# The Effective Management of Headache

*Other titles in the UK Key Advances in Clinical Practice Series*

The Effective Management of Benign Prostatic Disease and Lower Urinary Tract Symptoms

The Effective Management of Cancer Pain

The Effective Management of Metastatic Colorectal Cancer

The Effective Management of Ovarian Cancer

The Effective Management of Post-Operative Nausea and Vomiting

# The Effective Management of Headache

*Edited by*

Peter J Goadsby MD PhD DSc FRACP FRCP
*Professor of Clinical Neurology, National Hospital for Neurology
and Neurosurgery, Queen Square, London, UK*

Andrew J Dowson MB BS MRCGP
*General Practitioner and Director, King's College
Hospital Headache Service, London, UK*

Andrew Miles MSc MPhil PhD
*UeL Professor of Health Services Research and UK Key Advances
Series Organiser at St Bartholomew's Hospital, London, UK*

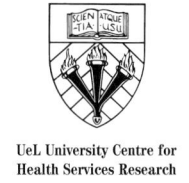

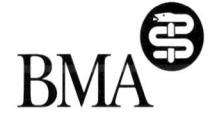

AESCULAPIUS MEDICAL PRESS
LONDON  SAN FRANCISCO  SYDNEY

Published by

Aesculapius Medical Press (London, San Francisco, Sydney)
UeL University Centre for Health Services Research
St Bartholomew's Hospital
London
EC1A 7BE

© Aesculapius Medical Press 1999

First published 1999

All rights reserved. No part of this publication may be reproduced or transmitted in any form or by any means, electronically or mechanically, including photocopying, recording or any other information storage or retrieval system, without prior permission in writing from the publishers.

British Library Cataloguing in Publication Data
A catalogue record for this book is available from the British Library

ISBN 1 903044 03 0

While the advice and information in this book are believed to be true and accurate at the time of going to press, neither the authors nor the publishers nor the sponsoring institutions can accept any legal responsibility or liability for any errors or omissions that may be made. In particular (but without limiting the generality of the preceding disclaimer) every effort has been made to check drug usages; however, it is possible that errors have been missed. Furthermore, dosage schedules are constantly being revised and new side-effects recognised. For these reasons, the reader is strongly urged to consult the drug companies' printed instructions before administering any of the drugs recommended in this book.

*Further copies of this volume are available from:*

Claudio Melchiorri
Research Dissemination Fellow
UeL Centre for Health Services Research
St Bartholomew's Hospital
London EC1 7BE

Fax: 0171 601 7085
e-mail: c.melchiorri@mds.qmw.ac.uk

Typeset, printed and bound in Britain by
Peter Powell Origination & Print Limited

# Contents

| | | |
|---|---|---|
| *List of contributors* | | *vi* |
| *Preface* | | *vii* |
| **Part 1 Evidence and assessment** | | 1 |
| 1 | The epidemiology and economics of headache<br>Kim Price | 3 |
| 2 | Differential diagnosis: what type of headache? When and how to investigate<br>Ra'ad Shakir | 23 |
| 3 | When to refer: a primary care perspective<br>Manuela Fontebasso | 31 |
| 4 | When to refer: a secondary care perspective<br>Richard Peatfield | 41 |
| 5 | Psychiatric perspectives of headache<br>Geir Madland and Charlotte Feinmann | 49 |
| **Part 2 Evidence and treatment** | | 61 |
| 6 | Treatment of headache and prophylaxis<br>Andrew J Dowson | 63 |
| 7 | Clinical effectiveness of migraine therapy: the number needed to treat and therapeutic gain calculations as emerging methods of evaluation<br>Peter J Goadsby | 77 |
| 8 | Cost-effectiveness of migraine therapy: evaluating new acute treatments using the example of the triptans<br>David Millson, Harry Ward, Wendy Clark and Martin Frischer | 93 |
| 9 | Investigation and management of migraine in women<br>Anne MacGregor | 107 |
| 10 | Investigation and management of migraine in children<br>John Wilson | 123 |
| 11 | The place and efficacy of complementary therapies<br>Tom Whitmarsh | 135 |
| *Index* | | *155* |

# Contributors

Wendy Clark BPharm MRPharmS, Lecturer, Department of Medicines Management, Keele University, Staffordshire, UK

Andrew J Dowson MB BS MRCGP, General Practitioner and Director, King's College Hospital Headache Service, London, UK

Charlotte Feinmann MSc MD FRCPsych FDS (Hon), Senior Lecturer, Academic Department of Psychiatry and Behavioural Sciences, University College, London, and Honorary Consultant Liaison Psychiatrist, Eastman Dental Hospital and Institute, London, UK

Manuela Fontebasso MB ChB, General Practitioner, Acomb, York, and Clinical Assistant, Headache Clinic, York District Hospital, York, UK

Martin Frischer BA PhD, Senior Lecturer, Department of Medicines Management, Keele University, Staffordshire, UK

Peter J Goadsby MD PhD DSc FRACP FRCP, Professor of Clinical Neurology, National Hospital for Neurology and Neurosurgery, London, UK

Anne MacGregor MB BS DFFP, Senior Registrar, The City of London Migraine Clinic, London, and Department of Gynaecology, St Bartholomew's Hospital, London, UK

Geir Madland BSc FDS RCS, MRC Research Fellow, Academic Department of Psychiatry and Behavioural Sciences, University College, London, and Honorary Registrar in Oral Medicine, Eastman Dental Hospital and Institute, London, UK

David Millson MD PhD FFPM, Professor of Medicines Management, Department of Medicines Management, Keele University, Staffordshire, UK

Richard Peatfield MD FRCP, Consultant Neurologist, Charing Cross Hospital, London, UK

Kim Price BSc MPhil, Senior Health Economist, GlaxoWellcome Research and Development, Greenford, Middlesex, UK

Ra'ad Shakir FRCP, Consultant Neurologist, Charing Cross Hospital, London, UK

Harry Ward BA MSc, Lecturer, Department of Medicines Management, Keele University, Staffordshire, UK

Tom Whitmarsh MA MRCP MFHom, Consultant Physician, Glasgow Homoeopathic Hospital, Glasgow, Scotland, UK

John Wilson PhD FRCP FRCPCH, Honorary Consultant Paediatric Neurologist, Great Ormond Street Hospital, London, UK

# Preface

Headache is among the commonest of clinical problems and its optimal effective management is a challenge as the field advances. This volume sets out a broad range of key advances, seeking to provide the reader with a wide update on largely clinically focused topics. Many of the chapters use advances in migraine, both therapeutic and non-therapeutic, to illustrate the principles.

The volume first examines the broad issues of the burden of headache: this takes the clinical form that we all see and the important health economic dimension which, although less obvious, must be considered, given that the total cost of headache to society runs into approximately $US8 billion per year.

On the clinical side, the differential diagnosis and referral of patients are covered from both the secondary and primary care perspectives and this provides interesting contrasts and insights.

Management issues are dealt with from both the pharmacotherapeutic and psychiatric dimensions. Prophylaxis is explicitly covered, while acute attack medications are reviewed in terms of summary measures and with an eye to cost. The number-needed-to-treat (NNT) analysis and therapeutic gain have been much discussed and, in the absence of head-to-head controlled trials, provide some limited way of comparing drugs.

The special topics of headache in women and in children are covered in individual chapters, and a comprehensive review of complementary treatments completes the broad canvas that is being addressed in the book.

In the current age, where doctors and health professionals are increasingly overwhelmed by clinical information, we have aimed to provide a fully current, fully referenced text which is as succinct as possible but as comprehensive as necessary. Neurologists and general practitioners will find it of particular use of part of their continuing medical education and specialist training, and we advance it explicitly as an excellent tool for these purposes. We anticipate, however, that the book will prove of not inconsiderable use to other members of the primary health care team, hospital neurology nurses and pharmacists as a reference text, and to commissioners of health services as the basis for discussion and negotiation of health contracts with their practising colleagues.

In conclusion, we thank Glaxo Wellcome UK for the grant of educational sponsorship which helped organise a national symposium held with the department of medical education of the British Medical Association at BMA House, at which synopses of the constituent chapters of this book were presented. Editing has been done for consistency, but the opinions expressed are those of individual chapter authors. We also thank The Migraine Trust (Registered Charity No. 244250) for its generous assistance in enabling a copy of this text to be placed in every hospital library in the UK.

*Peter J Goadsby* MD PhD DSc FRACP FRCP
*Andrew J Dowson* MB BS MRCGP
*Andrew Miles* MSc MPhil PhD

PART 1

# Evidence and Assessment

Chapter 1

# The epidemiology and economics of headache

*Kim Price*

## Introduction

It has long been known that headache is a common and often disabling condition (Olesen *et al.* 1993), but the true magnitude of headache as a health problem did not become apparent until the 1960s. Data from the early 1980s show headache to be one of the most common medical disorders, accounting at that time for more than 10 million visits to general practitioners each year in the USA alone (Cypress 1981). Many of these patients had suffered from chronic daily headaches for months or even years, with a clinical picture often attributed to 'tension', 'stress' or 'depression'.

## Epidemiology

From an epidemiological perspective, headache is a multifaceted phenomenon. It can be a manifestation of acute systemic or cranial infection, intracranial tumour, head injury, severe hypertension, cerebral hypoxia, and many diseases of the eye, nose, throat, teeth and ear. However, these conditions account for only a small number of headaches; most patients present with headache caused by muscular tension, migraine, or with head pain for which no structural cause is apparent (Berkow 1992). Headache has several determinants (e.g. genetic, physicochemical and stress-related) and effects (e.g. physiological and interpersonal), and presents a problem in terms of numbers of patients, the persistence of the condition, and the emotional pressure laid by patients upon families, friends and carers as a result of chronic pain (Barnat & Lake 1983).

Investigation of the epidemiology of headache helps to address a number of important concerns, including the true scope of the problem, the distribution of the disorder, the spectrum of severity and disability, patterns of diagnosis and therapy, and identification of diagnostic improvements and optimum treatments.

The exact prevalence of headache has long been debated. A number of studies carried out predominantly in the 1970s and 1980s estimated the prevalence in selected populations (e.g. general practice and hospital patients, school-children and various occupational groups) (Waters 1972, 1974a; Dalsgaard-Nielsen & Ulrich 1973; Philips 1977; Dhopesh *et al.* 1979; Ogunyemi 1984; Schwartz *et al.* 1997) as well as in the general population (Brewis *et al.* 1966; Waters 1970, 1974b; Crisp *et al.* 1977; Nikiforow & Hokkanen 1978; Hollnagel & Nørrelund 1980; D'Alessandro *et al.* 1988; Mendizabal & Rothrock 1998). Population-based studies are important for accurate definition of the epidemiology of headache, as only a small proportion of headache sufferers seek medical assistance (Sheftell 1997). Despite this, most studies are carried out in the clinic setting, even though fewer than 15 per cent of patients ever consult a neurologist and fewer than 2 per cent are seen by a headache specialist (Silberstein & Lipton 1996). Population-based studies circumvent the problems caused by selection bias under these circumstances.

The major problem in the study of the epidemiology of headache has been the classification of the numerous kinds of headache (Olesen *et al.* 1993; Hopkins 1996). Headache is a subjective complaint with no laboratory correlates, and diagnosis and classification are therefore reliant on information given by patients about their symptoms (Rasmussen 1995). Early classification systems tended to provide descriptions rather than operational definitions, and often posed significant problems in terms of the establishment of diagnostic validity. These difficulties were particularly apparent in the differentiation of migraine and tension headaches. For example, the classification system of the Ad Hoc Committee of the National Institute of Neurological Diseases and Blindness (NINDB) defined migraine as 'recurrent attacks of headache ... commonly unilateral in onset; are usually associated with anorexia and sometimes with nausea and vomiting; in some are preceded by, or associated with, conspicuous neurological and mood disturbances' (Ad Hoc Committee on Classification of Headache 1962). This (and the accompanying definition of tension or muscle contraction headache) are vague: terms such as 'recurrent' and 'commonly' are not defined, and the criteria are open to varied interpretation (Lipton & Stewart 1993a).

Difficulties in classifying headache are compounded by the episodic nature of the condition. The type of headache experienced may vary from attack to attack and from one time period to another in the same individual. Despite the observation that many patients suffer from more than one type of headache within the same period (e.g. migraine without aura and episodic tension-type headache), it has been common practice to categorise patients as having either one type of headache or another (i.e. migraine or tension headache). Because of this episodic and periodic variation, it is important to define clearly the time period over which prevalence is being studied. Population-based studies tend to assess lifetime experience of headache or one-year recall intervals. Lifetime history provides the broadest picture of each patient's headache experience, but such histories are generally considered to be reported with poor accuracy. The one-year recall interval, however, is considered to be more reliable for the overall assessment of headaches currently being experienced (Stewart & Lipton 1993).

Problems caused by the lack of precise, unambiguous and operational classification systems to aid in the study of headache led to the introduction in 1988 of explicit diagnostic criteria by the Headache Classification Committee of the International Headache Society (IHS) (1988). The IHS divides headaches into two broad groups:

- *primary,* in which the headache disorder itself is the underlying problem;
- *secondary,* in which the headache is symptomatic of an underlying condition.

The classification is hierarchical and consists of 13 diagnostic groups that are subdivided to allow for coding up to a 4-digit level. Ambiguous criteria are avoided, and it is possible to use the classification at different levels of sophistication. Importantly, the IHS system has been validated in clinic patients (Iversen *et al.* 1990) and has been shown to be applicable to random samples from the general population (Breslau *et al.* 1991; Rasmussen *et al.* 1991a; Pryse-Phillips *et al.* 1992; Stewart *et al.* 1992). The general categories of headache in the IHS scheme are shown in Table 1.1; a more detailed description of the two most extensively investigated and reported types, migraine and tension-type headache, and examples of diagnostic criteria are given in Tables 1.2 and 1.3, respectively.

## Prevalence

The difficulties described in classification and diagnosis of headache have contributed to strikingly different estimates of headache prevalence in various studies conducted in a number of countries. Several of these studies (from the USA and Western Europe) are summarised in Figure 1.1, and show the overall prevalence figure to vary from a relatively low 35 per cent to as much as nearly 100 per cent. It should be noted that in most studies the term 'headache' was not defined; in others (Ziegler *et al.* 1977; Rasmussen *et al.* 1991b), 'headache' was stated clearly to include all forms (migraine, tension-type, mild and severe, etc.).

Prevalence estimates may be heavily influenced by the way in which questions asked of patients in such studies are phrased. Some questionnaires ask: 'Do you suffer from headache?'; others ask: 'Do you have headache?' Interestingly, use of the words 'suffer from' appears to result in lower prevalence estimates than 'have'. Nevertheless, it is clear overall from research that headache is a widespread and common problem. The Nuprin Pain Report, a national epidemiological survey of the prevalence of headache and six other painful conditions that was conducted in 1,254 patients in the USA, showed a prevalence of headache of 78 per cent among women and 68 per cent among men (Taylor 1985). A larger survey (n=4,753) carried out in Denmark showed headache to be one of the most frequently reported disorders in the adult population, being more frequent than the common cold (Rasmussen *et al.* 1987). Most studies appear to show one-year or lifetime prevalence rates of at least 70 per cent for headache; indeed, a German survey (using IHS classification) of 4,061 individuals showed lifetime prevalence rates of over 90 per cent for both men and women (Göbel *et al.* 1994).

## Sex and age distribution

Inspection of the study results in Figure 1.1 shows that headache occurs more frequently in women than in men. This is partly caused by a high prevalence of migraine in women. However, tension-type headaches (together with several other types) are also more prevalent in women (Rasmussen *et al.* 1991b). This high relative

**6** Evidence and assessment

**Table 1.1** Major categories (with commonly encountered examples of subclassifications to the second level) of headache in the International Headache Society (IHS) classification

*Primary headache*

| | | |
|---|---|---|
| 1 | Migraine | 1.1 Migraine without aura |
| | | 1.2 Migraine with aura |
| 2 | Tension-type headache | 2.1 Episodic tension-type headache |
| | | 2.2 Chronic tension-type headache |
| 3 | Cluster headache & chronic paroxysmal hemicrania | 3.1 Cluster headache |
| 4 | Miscellaneous headaches unassociated with structural lesion | 4.1 Idiopathic stabbing headache |
| | | 4.2 External compression headache |
| | | 4.3 Cold stimulus headache |
| | | 4.4 Benign cough headache |
| | | 4.5 Benign exertional headache |
| | | 4.6 Headache associated with sexual activity |

*Secondary headache*

Headache associated with:

5  Head trauma
6  Vascular disorders
7  Non-vascular intracranial disorders
8  Substances or their withdrawal
9  Non-cephalic infection
10 Metabolic disorders
11 Headache or facial pain associated with disorder of the cranium, neck, eyes, ears, nose, sinuses, teeth, mouth or other facial or cranial structures
12 Cranial neuralgias
13 Headache not classifiable

*Source:* Headache Classification Committee of the International Headache Society (1988)

frequency of headache in women has been attributed partly to the influence of female hormones (Welch *et al.* 1984).

The prevalence of headache decreases after middle age, with many individuals becoming headache-free with increasing age (Granella *et al.* 1998). However, it is difficult to draw longitudinal conclusions from cross-sectional data. Lifetime prevalence data might be expected to show a cumulative trend of increasing prevalence with

**Table 1.2** Grouping of migraine and tension-type headaches according to the International Headache Society (IHS) classification

*1 Migraine*

1.1 Migraine without aura
1.2 Migraine with aura
1.3 Ophthalmoplegic migraine
1.4 Retinal migraine
1.5 Childhood periodic syndromes that may be precursors to or associated with migraine
1.6 Complications of migraine
1.7 Migrainous disorders not fulfilling the above criteria

*2 Tension-type headache*

| | |
|---|---|
| 2.1 Episodic tension-type headache | 2.1.1 Episodic tension-type headache associated with disorder of pericranial muscles |
| | 2.1.2 Episodic tension-type headache not associated with disorder of pericranial muscles |
| 2.2 Chronic tension-type headache | 2.2.1 Chronic tension-type headache associated with disorder of pericranial muscles |
| | 2.2.2 Chronic tension-type headache not associated with disorder of pericranial muscles |
| 2.3 Headache of the tension-type not fulfilling above criteria | |

*Source:* Headache Classification Committee of the International Headache Society (1988)

increasing age, but in, for example, two notable studies from the USA (Ziegler *et al.* 1977) and Denmark (Rassmussen *et al.* 1991b), lower lifetime prevalences of headache were reported by older patients. Poor memory and inaccurate answering may have played a role in these observations; additional explanations may include greater frequency of headaches in younger patients and naturally increased mortality rates in older headache sufferers. It is possible that headache prevalence in the older patient groups had never been as high as that seen in the present generation of younger patients. However, the hypothesis that mortality plays a part through elimination of greater numbers of older headache sufferers was refuted in a long-term follow-up study (Waters *et al.* 1983).

**Table 1.3** Diagnostic criteria for migraine without aura and for tension-type headache

*Diagnostic criteria for migraine without aura:*

A. At least 5 attacks fulfilling B–D

B. Attacks lasting 4–72 hours

C. Headache has at least 2 of the following characteristics:
- unilateral location
- pulsating quality
- moderate-to-severe intensity (inhibits or prohibits daily activities)
- aggravated by walking stairs or similar routine physical activity

D. During headache at least 1 of the following:
- nausea and/or vomiting
- photo- and phonophobia

*Diagnostic criteria for episodic tension-type headache:*

A. At least 10 previous headache episodes fulfilling criteria B–D below. Number of days with such headache <180/year.

B. Headache lasting from 30 minutes to 7 days.

C. At least 2 of the following pain characteristics:
- pressing/tightening (non-pulsating quality)
- mild-to-moderate intensity
- bilateral location
- no aggravation by walking stairs or similar routine physical activity

D. Both of the following:
- no nausea or vomiting (anorexia may occur)
- photo- and phonophobia are absent, or one but not the other is present

*Source:* Headache Classification Committee of the International Headache Society (1988)

One-year recall data also show lower headache prevalence rates in older than in younger patients (Waters 1974b; Newland *et al.* 1978; Nikiforow & Hokkanen 1978). Possible explanations for the lower prevalence with increasing age in these studies include:

- remission of headache with advancing age;
- increasing frequency of headache in younger age groups;

- a combination of the above two factors;
- more effective treatment in the elderly because of higher rates of medical consultation;
- recall bias in the elderly.

Age of onset data indicate that *de novo* cases of headache are infrequent in patients who have passed their middle years (Ziegler *et al.* 1977). Thus, some headache types may indeed be self-limiting. However, longitudinal follow-up studies are needed to distinguish true age-related effects from cohort or period effects.

## Socioeconomic factors

Many of the available socioeconomic data on headache are derived from patients with migraine and/or tension-type headache, and marital status, cohabitation, level of education, occupational category and employment status have not been associated in univariate or multivariate analyses with either of these headache types (Rasmussen 1992). Prevalence of headache seems also to be uniform across various social groups; although some studies in the past have suggested that migraine is more prevalent in persons of higher intelligence and/or social status (Nikiforow & Hokkanen 1978; D'Alessandro *et al.* 1988; Duckro *et al.* 1989; Merikangas *et al.* 1990), this may simply be a long-held clinical impression based on selection bias. Indeed Waters (1971) failed to find an association between migraine and social class or intelligence in a study using intelligence testing and occupation as measures of socioeconomic status, and other major studies have shown an inverse relationship between migraine prevalence and income (Lipton & Stewart 1993b; Stang & Osterhaus 1993).

## Specific headache types

Lifetime prevalence data for the primary headaches (to the 2-digit level) in a general population of 740 respondents are summarised in Table 1.4, and show the high prevalence of tension-type headache, migraine and cold stimulus headache relative to other types (Rasmussen & Olesen 1992).

Estimates of migraine prevalence, based largely on US and European data, vary widely, probably because of differences in definition of migraine and age and gender distributions (Green 1977; Jones & Harrop 1980; Bryn 1983; Henry *et al.* 1991; Wong *et al.* 1995). However, good agreement has been obtained in two major studies of one-year migraine prevalence: Rasmussen *et al.* (1991b) reported prevalence rates of 6 and 15 per cent in men and women, respectively; corresponding estimates in the US migraine study were 6 and 18 per cent (Stewart *et al.* 1992). The prevalence of migraine generally increases throughout childhood, adolescent and early adult life, peaks in the early 40s and declines thereafter. Before puberty, migraine is more prevalent in boys than in girls, but prevalence increases more rapidly in girls as adolescence approaches. The excess risk in women accumulates until mid-adult life and remains higher in women through to old age (which indicates that factors other than hormonal are involved) (Lipton & Stewart 1998).

**10** Evidence and assessment

The most common form of headache is the tension-type (chronic or episodic), with estimates of lifetime and one-year prevalence varying from around 30 to over 80 per cent (Waters 1972; Ziegler *et al.* 1977; Crisp *et al.* 1977; Nikiforow 1981; Rasmussen *et al.* 1991b). When considered separately, episodic tension-type headache has estimated one-year prevalence rates of 24–38 per cent, while the prevalence of chronic tension-type headache is 2–3 per cent (Lavados & Tenhamm 1998; Schwartz *et al.* 1998). As with migraine, prevalence is higher in women than in men and appears to decline with age (Waters 1972, 1974; Rasmussen *et al.* 1991b), but significant links with soecioeconomic factors have not been identified.

Notable among other headache types is cluster headache, a disorder much less extensively investigated and less well understood than migraine or tension-type headache. US data obtained via screening of over 6,400 patient records showed an overall age-adjusted incidence of 4.0 per 100,000 person-years for women and 15.6 per 100,000 person-years for men (Swanson *et al.* 1994). Peak incidence was in men aged 40–49 years and in women aged 60–69 years, with a significant link between smoking and cluster headache in men. Other estimates of prevalence include 90.0 per 100,000 in male military service candidates (Ekbom *et al.* 1978) and a calculated prevalence of 69.0 per 100,000 for the entire population of San Marino (D'Alessandro *et al.* 1986).

## Quality of life

The impact of headache on quality of life (QoL) of headache sufferers is underestimated, possibly because of the subjective nature of this disorder and the lack of reliable comparative measures (Solomon 1994). Generic QoL instruments, such as the

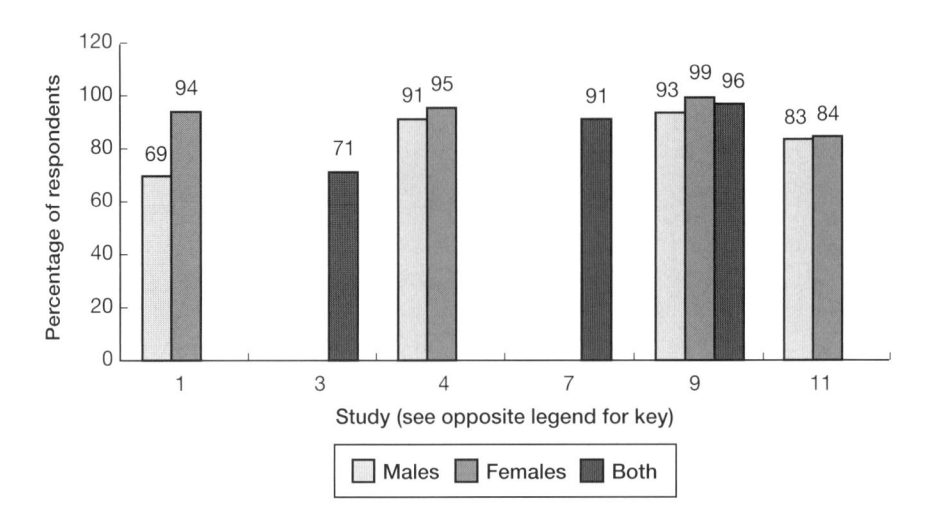

**Figure 1.1 (a)**

**(b)**

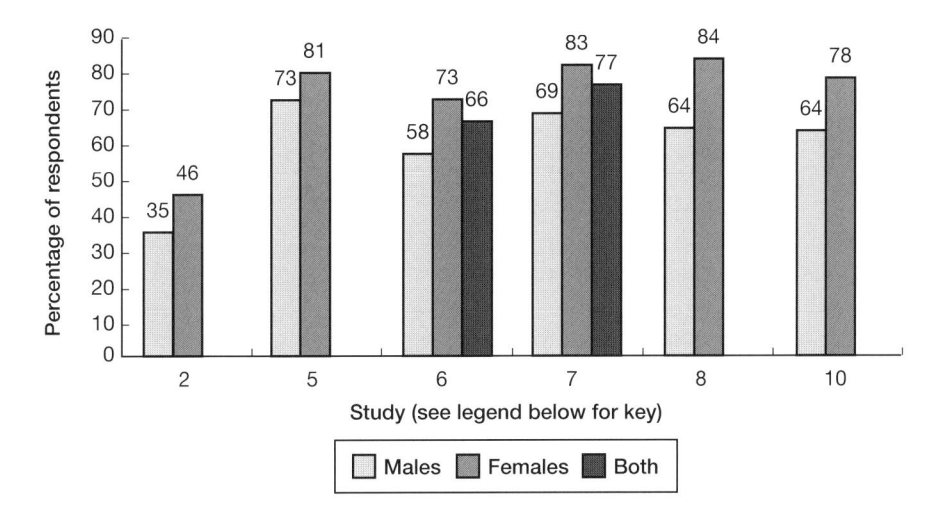

**Figure 1.1** Lifetime (a) and one-year (b) prevalence estimates of headache in Western European and US studies. All studies are general-population-based unless stated otherwise. Basic details of studies are given in the following table:

| Study (country) | No. of respondents | Age (years) |
| --- | --- | --- |
| 1 Crisp et al. 1977 (UK) | n=727 | Adults |
| 2 D'Alessandro et al. 1988 (Italy) | n=1144 | 7 yrs |
| 3 Göbel et al. 1994 (Germany) | n=4,061 | 18 yrs |
| 4 Linet et al. 1989 (USA) | n=10,169 | 12–29 yrs |
| 5 Newland et al. 1978 (UK) | n=2,066 | >18 yrs |
| 6 Nikiforow & Hokkanen 1978 (Finland) | n=3,067 | >15 yrs |
| 7 Nikiforow 1981 (Finland) | n=200 | >15 yrs |
| 8 Post & Gubbels 1986 (Netherlands) | n=2,252 (general practice patients) | 16–65 yrs |
| 9 Rasmussen et al. 1991b (Denmark) | n=740 | 25–64 yrs |
| 10 Waters 1974b (UK) | n=1,718 | >21 yrs |
| 11 Ziegler et al. 1977 (USA) | n=1,809 (church congregations) | >15 yrs |

**12** Evidence and assessment

**Table 1.4** Lifetime prevalence of primary headaches (IHS classification) in a general population of 740 respondents aged 25–64 years

| IHS classification | Percentage of responders |
| --- | --- |
| 1.1 Migraine without aura | 9 |
| 1.2 Migraine with aura | 6 |
| 2.1 Episodic tension-type headache | 66 |
| 2.2 Chronic tension-type headache | 3 |
| 3.1 Cluster headache | 0.1 |
| 4.1 Idiopathic stabbing headache | 2 |
| 4.2 External compression headache | 4 |
| 4.3 Cold stimulus headache | 15 |
| 4.4 Benign cough headache | 1 |
| 4.5 Benign exertional headache | 1 |
| 4.6 Headache with sexual activity | 1 |

*Source:* Rasmussen & Olesen (1992)

Medical Outcomes Study (MOS) Short Form SF-20 and SF-36, have been used in patients with chronic headache and migraine, respectively (Osterhaus & Townsend 1991; Solomon *et al.* 1993). Both studies showed chronic headache disorders to cause much more morbidity and impairment of function than had previously been appreciated. Solomon *et al.* (1993) studied 208 patients attending a headache clinic and found the proportion with poor health to range from 21 per cent for social functioning to 71 per cent for physical functioning. Using a mailed SF-36 questionnaire, Osterhaus & Townsend (1991), in their study of 845 patients with migraine, showed substantially diminished functioning and well-being compared with the general population. Physical functioning and health perception were similar to those of patients with arthritis or diabetes, but role and social functioning, pain and mental health scores were lower than those for other chronic conditions, such as hypertension and ischaemic heart disease.

## The economics of headache

The epidemiological data reviewed above highlight the scale of the public health dimension of headache. Prevalence and incidence are high, and people of all ages worldwide are affected. Although associated with high rates of morbidity, headache is not a fatal disorder and has therefore been regarded by health care providers as less serious than many other conditions. This impression is reinforced by the fact that the majority of patients with headache treat themselves with over-the-counter medications rather than consult a physician (Sheftell 1997; Antonov & Isaacson 1998). Nevertheless, the evidence shows an impact on quality of life and productivity, and a substantial disease burden on patients, their families and society.

## Economic impact of headache

A number of studies have examined the direct and indirect costs of headache (Solomon & Price 1997). The economic burden of headache is great and has often been underestimated because of the 'hidden' indirect nature of much of the cost. The total cost of headache to society has been estimated to be approximately €10 billion ($US8 billion) per year (Leonardi *et al.* 1998). It should be noted that there is no single universally accepted method for estimating the cost of headache. One approach is to consider directly measurable costs alone, but this does not consider hidden costs associated with disability and is limited in that many patients with headache who would benefit from medical care do not receive it. A second approach is to describe the illness in terms of pain, disability and diminished quality of life without attempting to attach a cost to the consequences of the illness. A third option is to attempt to estimate the total cost of illness (COI). Many studies of the economic burden of headache have been of the COI variety: they provide information beyond usual measures of prevalence and morbidity and can help to establish research and treatment priorities. However, there is some concern over the relevance of information provided by this method, as it invariably attaches a monetary value to illness but does not provide the economic information needed to determine the best and most efficient way to manage it (Davey & Leeder 1992; Drummond 1992). Furthermore, COI studies do not indicate whether more resources need to be allocated to disease management.

A Danish epidemiological study of headache in the general population showed that of all patients in paid employment at the time of evaluation, 5 per cent had been absent from work because of migraine and 9 per cent because of tension-type headache in the previous year (Rasmussen *et al.* 1992). These figures are similar to those from Britain (Waters 1986) and Norway (Winnem 1992), but higher than those from Northern Finland (Nikiforow & Hokkanen 1979). Overall, the total number of workdays lost across Europe from migraine and tension-type headache in the general employed population has been estimated at 270 days per 1,000 persons per year. Indeed, headache accounts for approximately 20 per cent of all absenteeism due to sickness. The economic benefits that might accrue from accurate diagnosis and effective management of headache are underlined by estimated total annual costs of reduced or lost productivity accruing from migraine of as much as $US17.2 billion in the USA alone (see below).

## Cost of illness: migraine

The large majority of studies that have attempted to quantify the economic burden of headache have focused on migraine. All use the human capital approach, which measures the burden of illness in terms of its effect on the flow of goods and services. With this approach, direct and indirect costs must be accounted for, and the assumption is made that earnings are a valid measure of productivity. In addition, most economic studies in patients with migraine make only passing reference to direct medical costs.

Diseases such as migraine, although affecting quality of life, may lead to relatively modest economic burdens in terms of use of health care resources, either because there are few effective interventions or because they are not regarded by health care professionals as 'important' (Drummond 1992). This point was made by Osterhaus *et al.* (1992) in their major COI study of patients with migraine.

Estimates of the direct costs of migraine are relatively consistent across studies, with comparable levels of use of prescription and over-the-counter medications (Green 1977; Celentano *et al.* 1992; Osterhaus *et al.* 1992; Rasmussen *et al.* 1992; Edmeads *et al.* 1993; Stang & Osterhaus 1993). Estimated total annual direct costs of migraine (1993 values) are $US12 million in Sweden (Björk & Roos 1991), $US 43–46 million in the UK (Blau & Drummond 1991), $US300 million in The Netherlands (van Roijen *et al.* 1995) and $US9.5 billion in the USA (Streator & Shearer 1996). A breakdown of costs of medical service consumption (in 1986 $US), as estimated by Osterhaus *et al.* (1992), is shown in Figure 1.2. The consultation rate for migraine in the UK has been reported to be 12.8 consultations per 1,000 (Blau & Drummond 1991). In the same study, it was estimated that, of the money spent by the NHS on migraine patients (£5 per patient per annum), 68 per cent represented medication, 25 per cent physician's visits and 7 per cent hospitalisation costs. A report assessing resource allocation in the management of migraine in the UK also concluded that the direct costs of migraine to the NHS were very low (approximately £30 million per annum), and that hospital referrals were unlikely to add more than £1–2 million to the overall costs of migraine management within the NHS (Bosanquet & Zammit Lucia 1992).

Several migraine studies (Table 1.5) have reported substantial loss of workdays (Figure 1.3); variations in estimates are most likely caused by differences between surveys in the wording of questions and the sociodemographic characteristics of participants. The majority of these studies did not attach any monetary value to the number of workdays lost; however, two groups of investigators set out specifically to estimate the economic impact of migraine. Using estimated median daily earnings data for 1986, Osterhaus *et al.* (1992) calculated a mean cost per month of missed workdays of $US254 for men and $US143 for women, and mean reduced productivity costs of $US193–298 for men and $US97–143 for women. This was extrapolated to a total annual cost (for 1986) of migraine to employers of $US5.6–17.2 billion, depending on the estimate of prevalence used. In contrast, using data from the National Health Interview Survey (NHIS), Stang & Osterhaus (1993) estimated lost productivity at $US1.4 billion per year for approximately 6.2 million migraine sufferers who worked outside the home. The difference in estimated indirect COI is most likely a result of the disparate nature of the two populations studied: the NHIS relied on a single respondent from each household to describe the health status of all family members (which may have led to an underestimation of migraine prevalence), whereas a clinic population of migraine sufferers (with correspondingly severe manifestations of disease) was studied by Osterhaus *et al.* (1992). European estimates

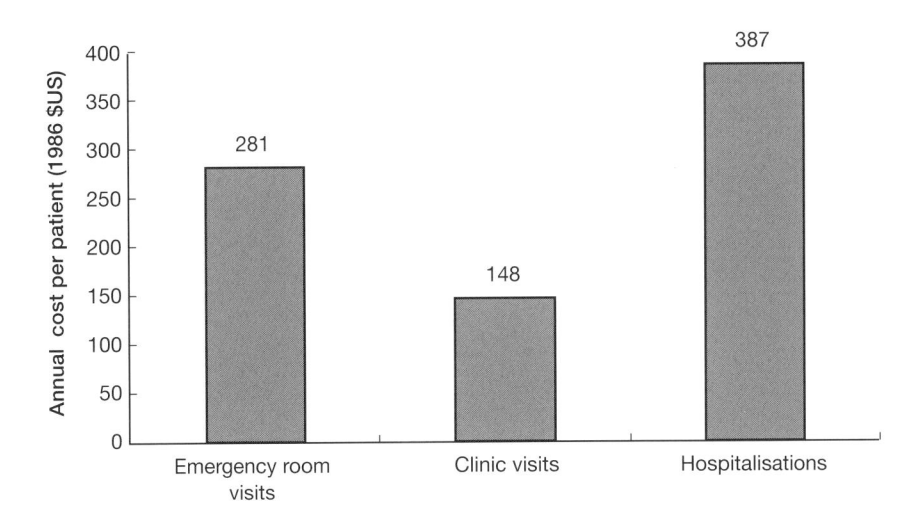

**Figure 1.2** Annual cost per patient of emergency room and clinic visits and hospitalisations in a clinic population of 648 patients with migraine (IHS criteria). The total annual direct medical cost for 648 patients was $US529,199 (Osterhaus et al. 1992)

over the last 12 years have put the total annual cost of productivity reduced or lost because of migraine at L.2,000 billion (£750 million) in Italy (Leonardi et al. 1998), L.500 million in San Marino (Benassi 1986), $US32 million in Sweden (Björk & Roos 1991), £611–741 million in the UK (Cull et al. 1992), $US1.2 billion in The Netherlands (van Roijen et al. 1995) and $US22 million in Turkey (Cankat 1991).

## Conclusions

The burden of headache to society is substantial. Although some misgivings over the relevance and utility of information provided by COI studies have been voiced in the literature (Davey & Leeder 1992; Drummond 1992), the available data show clearly that functioning of individuals with headache (usually reported as migraine) is significantly impaired. Clinical interventions should be matched to the severity of the disease. The goal of therapy should be to improve quality of life through reduced headache-related morbidity and to lower the high indirect cost of headache by reducing both absenteeism and decreased productivity at work.

Despite the prevalence and impact of headache, there are few published data on the effect of headache therapy on quality of life, outcomes or health care resource utilisation. Improvements in well-being were reported after abortive treatment with the non-steroidal anti-inflammatory drug (NSAID) diclofenac (Dahlöf & Björkman

**Table 1.5** Study details for 7 migraine cost of illness studies analysed in Figure 1.3

| Study | Population | Response method | Sample size | Migraine definition |
|---|---|---|---|---|
| 1 Childs & Sweetnam (1961) (UK) | Employee | In person | 1,607 | 'Symptom-based' |
| 2 Green (1977) (UK) | Mixed: employee/school | SAQ | 14,893 | 'Migraine' |
| 3 Jones & Harrop (1980) (UK) | Employee | Mail SAQ | 895 | Self-diagnosed |
| 4 Newland et al. (1978) (UK) | Community | In person | 2,065 | 2 of nausea, unilateral pain or warning |
| 5 Nikiforow & Hokkanen (1979)* (Finland) | Community | Mail SAQ | 200 | 'Vascular headache' |
| 6 Osterhaus et al. (1992) (US) | Clinic | Mail SAQ | 648 | IHS 1988 |
| 7 Rasmussen et al. (1992) (Denmark) | Community | In person | 740 | IHS 1988 |

\* Average No. days absent from work/school/regular activities per year per migraine sufferer
IHS = International Headache Society classification
SAQ = self-administered questionnaire

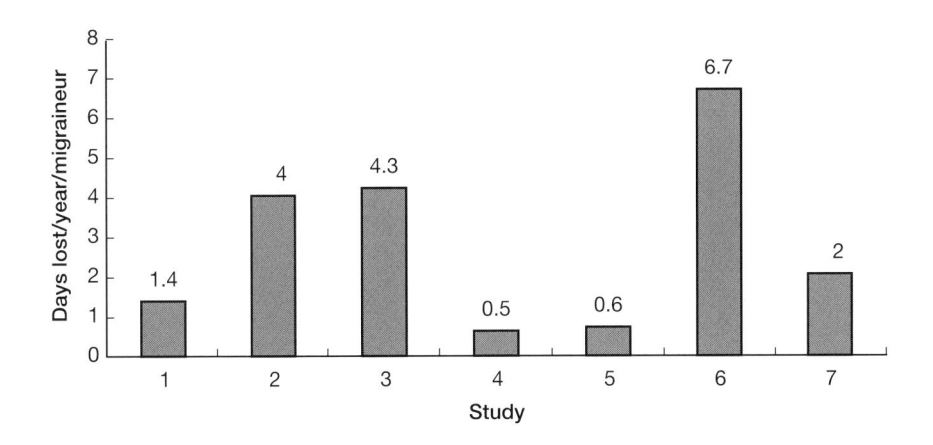

**Figure 1.3** Productivity losses associated with migraine. Average number of workdays lost per year per migraine sufferer in 7 cost of illness studies. Study details are shown in Table 1.5.

1993), and improved role functioning (ability to work) was documented in patients who received flurbiprofen, another NSAID, prophylactically (Solomon & Kunkel 1992). In recent years, much attention has focused on the use of novel serotonin 5-HT$_1$ agonists in the treatment of migraine. A number of US and European studies have shown the benefits of sumatriptan treatment in both improving the quality of life of migraine sufferers and reducing the indirect costs associated with migraine (Bosanquet & Zammit-Lucia 1992; Boureau *et al.* 1995; Adelman *et al.* 1996; Clarke *et al.* 1996; Cohen *et al.* 1996; Greiner & Addy 1996; Gross *et al.* 1996; Mushet *et al.* 1996; Streator & Shearer 1996; Cortelli *et al.* 1997; Dahlof *et al.* 1997; Ferrari 1998; Larbig & Brüggenjürgen 1997; Legg *et al.* 1997).

Thus, new opportunities for cost-effective intervention should lead to improvements in headache therapy and reductions in indirect costs. Valid and reliable tools are now available to assist researchers in understanding the effect of headache on patients' functioning and well-being, and the demonstration of improved outcomes will identify interventions that reduce headache-related morbidity and costs to society associated with lost productivity.

## *References*

Adelman J, Sharfman M, Johnson R *et al.* (1996). Impact of oral sumatriptan on workplace productivity and health-related quality of life, healthcare use, and patient satisfaction with medication in nurses with migraine. *American Journal of Managed Care* **2**, 1407–16.

Ad Hoc Committee on Classification of Headache (1962). Classification of headache. *Journal of the American Medical Association* **179**, 717–8.

Antonov K & Isaacson D (1998). Headache and analgesia use in Sweden. *Headache* **38**, 97–104.

Barnat M R & Lake III A E (1983). Patient attitudes about headache. *Headache* **23**, 229–37.

Benassi G (1986). The economic burden of headache: an epidemiological study in the Republic of San Marino. *Headache* **26**, 457–9.

Berkow R (ed.) (1992). *Merck manual of diagnosis and therapy* 16th edn. Merck Research Laboratories, Rahway (NJ).

Björk S & Roos P (1991). *Economic aspects of migraine in Sweden.* Institute for Health Economics, Lund, Sweden.

Blau J N & Drummond M F (1991). *Migraine.* Office of Health Economics, London.

Bosanquet N & Zammit Lucia J (1992). Migraine – a strategy for treatment. *Health Policy Review.* Paper No.1.

Bosanquet N & Zammit-Lucia J (1992). Migraine: prevention or cure? *British Journal of Medical Economics* **2**, 81–91.

Boureau F & the French Sumatriptan Study Group (1995). Comparison of subcutaneous sumatriptan with usual acute treatments for migraine. *European Neurology* **35**, 264–9.

Breslau N, Davis C C & Andreski P (1991). Migraine, psychiatric disorders and suicide attempts: an epidemiologic study of young adults. *Psychiatry Research* **37**, 11–23.

Brewis M, Poskanzer D C, Rolland C *et al.* (1966). Neurological disease in an English city. *Acta Neurologica Scandinavica* **42** (Suppl.24), 1–89.

Bryn G W (1983). Epidemiology of migraine: a personal view. *Headache* **23**, 127–33.

Cankat F (1991). Headache prevalence in Turkish women. In *New advances in headache research 2* (ed. F Clifford Rose). Smith-Gordon & Co. Ltd, London.

Celentano D D, Stewart W F, Lipton R B *et al.* (1992). Medication use and disability among migraineurs: a national probability sample survey. *Headache* **32**, 223–8.

Childs A J & Sweetnam M T (1961). A study of 104 cases of migraine. *Brit J Industr Med* **18**, 234–6.

Clarke C E, MacMillan L, Sondhi S *et al.* (1996). Economic and social impact of migraine. *Quarterly Journal of Medicine* **89**, 77–84.

Cohen J A, Beall D G, Miller D W *et al.* (1996). Subcutaneous sumatriptan for the treatment of migraine: humanistic, economic and clinical consequences. *Family Medicine* **28**, 171–7.

Cortelli P, Dahlöf C, Bouchard J *et al.* (1997). A multinational investigation of the impact of subcutaneous sumatriptan. III. Workplace productivity and non-workplace activity. *Pharmacoeconomics* **11** (Suppl.1), 35–42.

Crisp A H, Kalucy R S, McGuinness B *et al.* (1977). Some clinical, social and psychological characteristics of migraine subjects in the general population. *Postgraduate Medical Journal* **53**, 691–7.

Cull R E, Wells N E J & Miocevich M L (1992). The economic cost of migraine. *British Journal of Medical Economics* **2**, 103–15.

Cypress B K (1981). *Patients' reasons for visiting physicians; national ambulatory medical care survey. Vital and Health Statistics*, Series 13, No. 56, DHHS publication No. 82–1717, US Government Printing Office, Washington (DC).

Dahlöf C, Bouchard J, Cortelli P *et al.* (1997). A multinational investigation of the impact of subcutaneous sumatriptan. II. Health-related quality of life. *Pharmacoeconomics* **11** (Suppl.1), 24–34.

D'Alessandro R, Gamberini G, Benassi G *et al.* (1986). Cluster headache in the Republic of San Marino. *Cephalalgia* **6**, 159–62.

D'Alessandro R, Benassi G, Lenzi P L *et al.* (1988). Epidemiology of headache in the Republic of San Marino. *Journal of Neurology, Neurosurgery and Psychiatry* **51**, 21–7.

Dalsgaard-Nielsen T & Ulrich J (1973). Prevalence and heredity of migraine and migranoid headaches among 461 Danish doctors. *Headache* **12**, 168–72.

Davey P J & Leeder S R (1992). The cost of migraine: more than just a headache? *Pharmacoeconomics* **2**, 5–7.

Dhopesh V, Anwar R & Herring C (1979). A retrospective assessment of emergency department patients with complaint of headache. *Headache* **19**, 37–42.

Drummond M (1992). Cost of illness studies: a major headache? *Pharmacoeconomics* **2**, 1–4.

Duckro P N, Tait R C & Margolis R B (1989). Prevalence of very severe headache in a large US metropolitan area. *Cephalalgia* **9**, 199–205.

Edmeads J, Findlay H, Tugwell P *et al.* (1993). Impact of migraine and tension-type headache on lifestyle, consulting behaviour, and medication use: a Canadian population survey. *Canadian Journal of Neurological Science* **20**, 131–7.

Ekbom K, Ahlborg B & Schele R (1978). Prevalence of migraine and cluster headache in Swedish men of 18. *Headache* **18**, 9–19.

Ferrari M D (1998). The economic burden of migraine to society. *Pharmacoeconomics* **13**, 667–76.

Göbel H, Petersen-Braun M & Soyka D (1994). The epidemiology of headache in Germany: a nationwide survey of a representative sample on the basis of the headache classification of the International Headache Society. *Cephalalgia* **14**, 97–106.

Granella F, Cavallini A, Sandrini G *et al.* (1998). Long-term outcome of migraine. *Cephalalgia* **18** (Suppl.21), 30–3.

Green J E (1977). A survey of migraine in England 1975–1976. *Headache* **17**, 67–8.

Greiner D & Addy S N (1996). Sumatriptan use in a large group-model healthcare maintenance organisation. *American Journal of Health Systems Pharmacy* **53**, 633–8.

Gross M L P, Dowson A J, Deavy L *et al.* (1996). Impact of oral sumatriptan 50 mg on work productivity and quality of life in migraine. *British Journal of Medical Economics* **10**, 231–46.

Headache Classification Committee of the International Headache Society (1988). Classification and diagnostic criteria for headache disorders, cranial neuralgias and facial pain. *Cephalalgia* **8** (Suppl.7), 1–96.

Henry P, Michel P, Dartigues J F *et al.* (1991). Migraine prevalence in France. In *New advances in headache research 2* (ed. F Clifford Rose). Smith Gordon & Co. Ltd, London.

Hollnagel H & Nørrelund N (1980). Headache among 40-year-olds in Glostrup. *Ugeskr Laeger* **142**, 3071–7.

Hopkins A (1996). The epidemiology of headache and migraine, and its meaning for neurological services. *Schweizerische Medizinische Wochenschrift* **126**, 128–35.

Iversen H K, Langemeark M, Andersson P G *et al.* (1990). Clinical characteristics of migraine and episodic tension-type headache in relation to old and new diagnostic criteria. *Headache* **30**, 514–19.

Jones A & Harrop C (1980). Study of migraine and treatment of acute attacks in industry. *Journal of Medical Research* **8**, 321–5.

Larbig W & Brüggenjürgen B (1997). Work productivity and resource consumption among migraineurs under current treatment and during treatment with sumatriptan – an economic evaluation of acute treatment in moderate to severe migraineurs. *Headache Quarterly* **8**, 237–46.

Lavados P M & Tenhamm E (1998). Epidemiology of tension-type headache in Santiago, Chile: a prevalence study. *Cephalalgia* **18**, 552–8.

Legg R F, Sclar D A, Nemec N L *et al.* (1997). Cost-effectiveness of sumatriptan in a managed care population. *American Journal of Managed Care* **3**, 117–22.

Leonardi M, Musicco M & Nappi G (1998). Headache as a major public health problem: current status. *Cephalalgia* **18** (Suppl.21), 66–9.

Linet M S, Stewart W F, Celentano D D *et al.* (1989). An epidemiologic study of headache among adolescents and young adults. *Journal of the American Medical Association* **261**, 2211–16.

Lipton R B & Stewart W F (1993a). Reliability in headache diagnosis. *Cephalalgia* **13**, 29.

Lipton R B & Stewart W F (1993b). Migraine in the United States: epidemiology and health care use. *Neurology* **43** (Suppl.3), 6–10.

Lipton R B & Stewart W F (1998). Migraine headaches: epidemiology and comorbidity. *Clinical Neuroscience* **5**, 2–9.

Mendizabal J E & Rothrock J F (1998). An inter-regional comparative study of headache clinic populations. *Cephalalgia* **18**, 57–9.

Merikangas K R, Angst J & Isler H (1990). Migraine and psychopathology. *Archives of General Psychiatry* **47**, 849–53.

Mushet G R, Miller D, Clements B *et al.* (1996). Impact of sumatriptan on workplace nonwork activities and health-related quality of life among hospital employees with migraine. *Headache* **36**, 137–43.

Newland C A, Illis L S, Robinson P K *et al.* (1978). A survey of headache in an English city. *Research and Clinical Studies in Headache* **5**, 1–20.

Nikiforow R (1981). Headache in a random sample of 200 persons: a clinical study of a population in Northern Finland. *Cephalalgia* **1**, 99–107.

Nikiforow R & Hokkanen E (1978). An epidemiological study of headache in an urban and a rural population in northern Finland. *Headache* **18**, 137–45.

Nikiforow R & Hokkanen E (1979). Effects of headache on working ability, a survey of an urban and a rural population in Northern Finland. *Headache* **19**, 214–8.

Ogunyemi A O (1984). Prevalence of headache among Nigerian university students. *Headache* **24**, 127–30.

Olesen J, Tfelt-Hansen P & Welch KMA (eds) (1993). *The headaches*. Raven Press, New York.

Osterhaus J T & Townsend R J (1991). The quality of life of migraineurs. A cross-sectional profile. *Cephalalgia* **11** (Suppl.11), 103–4.

Osterhaus J T, Gutterman D L & Plachetka J R (1992). Healthcare resource and lost labour costs of migraine headache in the US. *Pharmacoeconomics* **2**, 67–76.

Philips C (1977). Headache in general practice. *Headache* **16**, 322–9.

Post D & Gubbels J W (1986). Headache: an epidemiological survey in a Dutch rural general practice. *Headache* **26**, 122–5.

Pryse-Phillips W, Findlay H, Tugwell P *et al.* (1992). A Canadian population survey in the clinical, epidemiologic and societal impact of migraine and tension-type headache. *Canadian Journal of Neurological Science* **19**, 333–9.

Rasmussen B K (1992). Migraine and tension-type headache in a general population: psychosocial factors. *International Journal of Epidemiology* **2**, 1138–43.

Rasmussen B K (1995). Epidemiology of headache. *Cephalalgia* **15**, 45–68.

Rasmussen B K & Olesen J (1992). Symptomatic and non-symptomatic headaches in a general population. *Neurology* **42**, 1225–31.

Rasmussen B K, Groth M V, Bredkjær S R *et al.* (1987). *Sundhed & Sygelighed i Danmark*. Dansk Institut for Klinisk Epidemiologi, Copenhagen.

Rasmussen B K, Jensen R & Olesen J (1991a). A population-based analysis of the diagnostic criteria of the International Headache Society. *Cephalalgia* **11**, 129–34.

Rasmussen B K, Jensen R, Schroll M *et al.* (1991b). Epidemiology of headache in a general population – a prevalence study. *Journal of Clinical Epidemiology* **44**, 1147–57.

Rasmussen B K, Jensen R & Olesen J (1992). Impact of headache on sickness absence and utilization of medical services: a Danish population study. *Journal of Epidemiology and Community Health* **42**, 443–6.

Schwartz B S, Stewart W F & Lipton R B (1997). Lost workdays and decreased work effectiveness associated with headaches in the workplace. *Journal of Occupational and Environmental Medicine* **39**, 320–7.

Schwartz B S, Stewart W F, Simon D *et al.* (1998). Epidemiology of tension-type headache. *Journal of the American Medical Association* **279**, 381–3.

Sheftell F D (1997). Role and impact of over-the-counter medications in the management of headache. *Neurologic Clinics* **15**, 187.

Silberstein S D & Lipton R B (1996). Headache epidemiology. Emphasis on migraine. *Neuroepidemiology* **14**, 421–34.

Solomon G D (1994). Quality-of-life assessment in patients with headache. *Pharmacoeconomics* **6**, 34–41.

Solomon G D & Kunkel R S (1992). Long-term use of flurbiprofen in migraine prophylaxis. *Headache* **32**, 269–70.

Solomon G D & Price K L (1997). Burden of migraine. A review of its socioeconomoc impact. *Pharmacoeconomics* **11** (Suppl.1), 1–10.

Solomon G D, Skobieranda F G & Gragg L A (1993). Quality of life and well being of headache patients: measurement by the Medical Outcomes Study Instrument. *Headache* **33**, 351–8.

Stang P E & Osterhaus J T (1993). Impact of migraine in the United States: data from the National Health Interview Survey. *Headache* **33**, 29–35.

Stewart W F & Lipton R B (1993). Societal impact of headache. In *The headaches* (ed. J Olesen, P Tfelt-Hansen & K M A Welch). Raven Press Limited, New York.

Stewart W F, Lipton R, Celentano D D *et al.* (1992). Prevalence of migraine headache in the United States. *Journal of the American Medical Association* **267**, 64–9.

Streator S E & Shearer S W (1996). Pharmacoeconomic impact of injectable sumatriptan on migraine-associated healthcare costs. *American Journal of Managed Care* **2**, 139–43.

Swanson J W, Yanagihara T, Stang P E *et al.* (1994). Incidence of cluster headaches: a population-based study in Olmsted County, Minnesota. *Neurology* **44**, 433–7.

Taylor H (ed) (1985). *The Nuprin pain report.* Louis Harris & Associates, New York.

van Roijen L, Essink-Bot M L, Koopmanschap M A *et al.* (1995). Societal perspective on the burden of migraine in the Netherlands. *Pharmacoeconomics* **7**, 170–9.

Waters W E (1970). Community studies of the prevalence of headache. *Headache* **9**, 178–86.

Waters W E (1971). Migraine: intelligence, social class, and familial prevalence. *British Medical Journal* **2**, 77–81.

Waters W E (1972). Headache and migraine in general practitioners. In *The migraine headache and dixarit: proceedings of a symposium held at Churchill College, Cambridge.* Boehringer Ingelheim, Bracknell, England, pp. 31–44.

Waters W E (1974a). *The epidemiology of migraine.* Boehringer Ingelheim, Bracknell, Oxford.

Waters W E (1974b). The Pontypridd headache survey. *Headache* **14**, 81–90.

Waters W E (1986). Headache. In *Series in clinical epidemiology* (ed. G J Bourke). Croom Helm, London & Sydney.

Waters W E, Campbell M J & Elwood P C (1983). Migraine, headache, and survival in women. *British Medical Journal* **287**, 1442–3.

Welch K M A, Darnley D & Simkins R T (1984). The role of estrogen in migraine: a review and hypothesis. *Cephalalgia* **4**, 227–36.

Winnem J (1992). Prevalence of adult migraine in general practice. *Cephalalgia* **12**, 300–3.

Wong T W, Wong K S, Yu T S *et al.* (1995). Prevalence of migraine and other headaches in Hong Kong. *Neuroepidemiology* **14**, 82–91.

Ziegler D K, Hassanein R S & Couch J R (1977). Characteristics of life headache histories in a nonclinic population. *Neurology* **27**, 265–9.

Chapter 2

# Differential diagnosis: what type of headache? When and how to investigate

*Ra'ad Shakir*

## Introduction

The vast majority of headaches do not need investigation. Taking a good history is the essence of diagnosis. When headache is recurrent, chronic and is associated with classical symptoms of tension-type headache or migraine, then investigations are hardly rewarding. This chapter presents an overview of the life-threatening causes of headaches. In these types of headaches secondary referral is essential and sophisticated neurological investigations, intensive care, neurosurgical expertise and hospital management are needed. The timely availability of expert advice on such cases remains a major issue in most general practices. Perhaps one needs to emphasise the importance of recognising danger signs and being able to act quickly to avert disaster.

## Subarachnoid haemorrhage

Acute severe headache which in most patients is described as the worst headache ever is always a danger sign which needs further evaluation. Subarachnoid haemorrhage is a cause of sudden severe headache and sudden death. It may follow exertion in a third of the cases. Associated other symptoms and signs include nausea, vomiting and neck stiffness, which may progress to unconsciousness. Epileptic seizures, photophobia and cranial nerve palsies, including third-nerve palsy, are well recognised. The classical syndrome of sudden severe headaches, vomiting, loss of consciousness, a third-nerve palsy with pupillary dilatation due to a bleed from a posterior communication artery aneurysm is well established.

The majority of patients with subarachnoid haemorrhage have a congenital aneurysm, others have an arteriovenous malformation (AVM) and the ratio varies in different populations: aneurysms are more likely in western populations, while AVMs are commoner in orientals. Subarachnoid haemorrhage can happen when blood leaks into the ventricles from an intracerebral bleed commonly seen in hypertension and this usually suggests a poor prognosis. Referring patients urgently to a hospital is essential. CT scanning, if done urgently within hours of the haemorrhage, will reveal blood in the subarachnoid space. The positivity of CT scanning diminishes with time and by the fourth day only 40 per cent of CT scans are positive (Adams *et al.* 1983).

A good story suggestive of subarachnoid haemorrhage, even without classical signs of neck stiffness or clouding of consciousness, merits close scrutiny. If the head

CT scan is positive for blood, lumbar puncture is not necessary. However, lumbar puncture is needed when the CT scan is negative or late, looking for uniformly blood-stained cerobrospinal fluid (CSF). After about 6–12 hours xanthochromia appears in the CSF. This may persist for 2–3 weeks. Angiography should be considered if the story of sudden severe headache is convincing in the absence of CT or even CSF evidence of a bleed. The term 'thunderclap headache' is defined as a headache starting within seconds, reaching a peak in a minute, with a normal CSF examination within 48 hours; it is rare in this type of presentation to find a ruptured berry aneurysm on full investigations, including angiography. Transferring patients to a specialised neurosurgical unit is essential and this should be done as soon as possible. Neurosurgeons will carry out formal angiography followed by either clipping or coiling aneurysms with platinum wire.

Aneurysms can be familial and it is always worthwhile investigating members of families where there have been at least two cases of subarachnoid haemorrhage previously. This has been shown to be a genetic condition and many asymptomatic patients have been found to have unruptured aneurysms (Ronkainen *et al.* 1997). There is still some controversy as to what to do for such individuals who are completely asymptomatic. Some evidence has shown that the size of aneurysms is essential: large aneurysms which are bigger than 1 cm in diameter will probably require prophylactic clipping or coiling because of a higher chance of bleeding, which outweighs the risks of treatment (International Study of Unruptured Intracranial Aneurysms Investigators 1998).

Screening individuals with a positive family history for aneurysmal subarachnoid haemorrhage or ruling out subarachnoid haemorrhage in suspicious acute headache patients can be done with MR angiography (MRA). This technique is now available in most major centres. Modern MR equipment is capable of visualising aneurysms in or around the circle of Willis non-invasively and without contrast injections. The technique is not completely infallible and although there are no formal studies, the accuracy is around 95 per cent. Minor leaking of blood from an aneurysm before a major bleed is known and this may be a cause for investigating sudden headaches.

## Arteriovenous malformations

The majority of AVMs are asymptomatic and are found incidentally on imaging for some other cause. AVMs usually present with epilepsy or intracerebral haemorrhage causing acute headache (Arteriovenuos Malformation Study Group 1999). They can, on rare occasions, cause headache if they are large and if the headache is persistently unilateral. Once discovered on CT scanning usually without and with contrast, then further investigations are needed in order to determine their size, arterial supply and venous drainage. Some large AVMs are fed from several intracranial arteries both in the carotid and the vertebral circulation and their drainage is so extensive to make them inoperable. The ideal treatment for AVMs remains surgical provided that removal of the AVM does not lead to any neurological deficit. Other methods of treatment include glue injection through an arteriogram and this has to be judged according to the size of the AVM. It has also to be done with great care in case the thrombosing part of the AVM may lead to an infarction in an eloquent area of the brain.

Some AVMs are suitable for stereotactic radiosurgery using the gamma ray knife. This technology employs radiotherapy with gamma rays from multiple sources, which concentrate in a single spot in the brain. The localised radiotherapy will very slowly lead to thrombosis of an AVM over some two years. During the time the AVM is slowly being obliterated, there is a chance of haemorrhage. One therefore has to judge the risks of this procedure versus other methods of treatment. The procedure is attractive because it is non-invasive, although the long-term prognosis of focal radiation over 10–20 years is not known.

With the use of MRI scanning, slow-flow cavernous angiomas are discovered regularly. They can either be an incidental finding or sometimes cause epileptic seizures. MRI nearly always shows a small area of haemosiderin around the cavernous angioma suggesting previous small blood leakage. Many of these angiomas can be left alone without any surgical intervention. Gamma ray knife use in this type of slow-flow angioma is not effective.

## Sexual headache

Headache during sexual intercourse is not uncommon and the term 'coital cephalalgia' is coined here. Individuals of both sexes complain of sudden severe occipital headache at the point of orgasm and this can last 20–30 minutes and then subsides slowly. In the vast majority of patients this is a benign condition but if it has occurred for the first time, it is worth investigating as any other severe exertional headache. The International Headache Society (1988) classification recognises three types:

- a dull ache intensifying as sexual excitement increases;
- an explosive type at orgasm;
- a postural type resembling low-pressure headache after coitus.

The explosive type is the one that is usually encountered in clinical practice. It is very difficult to put a figure on the chance that this headache may be due to an intracranial bleed from an aneurysm, but around 1 in 20 patients may have a haemorrhage causing this headache. If the headache has occurred for the first time with a normal neurological examination and the pain subsided within an hour or so, MR angiography can be performed to rule out the possibility of a sizable aneurysm. If, however, the pain has persisted for more than an hour or two, then perhaps one needs to treat this as a possible subarachnoid haemorrhage and the patient may need to be referred for CT scanning, possible lumbar puncture and formal angiography.

There is no clear evidence on how to treat patients with benign sexual headache; treatment with propranolol for three months is the accepted standard therapy (Silbert *et al.* 1990). These patients are usually very apprehensive and require reassurance.

## Dural sinus thrombosis

Intracranial venous sinuses can thrombose and cause headache with variable severity. If there is sagittal sinus as well as lateral sinus thrombosis, the headache can be severe and is associated with nausea, vomiting and bilateral papilloedema. These patients can also present with seizures and coma, depending on the severity of the thrombosis. If a single lateral sinus is thrombosed, chronic headache can be the presenting symptom and papilloedema may not be apparent. CT scanning is not very specific for this condition, although it may show some tell-tale signs. MRI of the brain, and more specifically MR venography, are quite adequate in diagnosis. Formal angiography is not necessary in most patients. Patients with sagittal or other intracranial sinus thrombosis need to be fully investigated for a possible cause of venous thrombosis and a thrombophilia screen is performed to rule out the possibility of a coagulation defect. Anticardiolipin antibodies, lupus anticoagulant, protein C and protein S deficiencies should be looked for. Immediate heparinisation and long-term warfarin are instituted in all patients. Treatment is usually continued for a year and then withdrawn.

## Increased intracranial pressure

Brain tumours, subdural haematomas, extradural haematomas and other causes of increased intracranial pressure will produce their own specific neurological symptoms and signs, and CT scanning has to be performed if there is any suspicion that this is the case. Perhaps this possibility is the main reason which drives patients to seek specialist advice and request scanning. For those patients who demand to be referred to a specialist to rule out a brain tumour, this is entirely acceptable and should be performed. The problem, however, is that in many district general hospitals CT scans are reported by general radiologists with little expertise in neuroradiology and in some patients with headache a dubious report will create more concern rather than solve a problem. Standard non-contrasted CT scans may miss intracranial tumours and, giving that IV contrast has a small risk of allergy, it requires radiologist supervision.

The yield of performing cranial MRI on all patients presenting with non-migranous headache with a normal neurological examination is 2.4 per cent, which is not insubstantial (Frishberg 1994). According to the Quality Standards Subcommittee of the American Academy of Neurology (1994), the routine use of neuroimaging is not warranted in adults with recurrent headaches that have been defined as migraine – including those with visual aura – with no recent change in pattern, no history of seizures and no other focal neurologic signs or symptoms. In patients with atypical headache patterns, a history of seizures, or focal neurologic signs or symptoms, CT or MRI may be indicated. While resources should always be used carefully, the possibility of missing a treatable intracranial cause for the headache should always be considered.

## Intracranial hypertension

Increased intracranial pressure without the presence of a space-occupying lesion or venous sinus thrombosis is termed 'benign intracranial hypertension' (BIH) or idiopathic intracranial hypertension. It can be a result of vitamin A toxicity, hypoparathyroidism, drug use, such as nalidixic acid, and steroid withdrawal. Other associated factors include severe anaemia and the use of tetracycline and the oral contraceptive pill – these, however, are controversial. In idiopathic cases BIH (pseudotumour cerebri) patients are usually obese young females presenting with headaches, transient visual obscuration and pulsatile tinnitus. Papilloedema in the absence of any other focal neurological sign is the classic presentation. The significant complications of BIH include loss of visual acuity and visual field. Careful ophthalmological assessment is essential to avoid permanent visual defect. There are rare cases of BIH without papilloedema reported. Management includes the use of acetozolamide, dexamethzone, and optic nerve sheath fenestration to relieve the pressure on the optic nerves. Lumboperitoneal shunting is of limited value.

## Intracranial hypotension

This condition is rare and is due to a dural tear. The most obvious cause is lumbar puncture or CSF leak owing to trauma or surgery. It can occur after severe exertion or sometimes *de novo*. Patients present with headache which is made worse by upright posture and relieved by lying flat. The headache is usually induced by performing a Valsalva manoeuvre while lying flat, which will help to confirm the clinical impression of a low-pressure orthostatic headache syndrome. Occult CSF rhinorrhoea and otorrhoea should be looked for. The pain is associated with a pulling sensation in the neck and what is described as an echo sound in both ears. If lumbar puncture is performed on such individuals, the CSF pressure is very low (less than 6 cm fluid). Brain MRI shows dural enhancement and diffuse mengingeal enhancement in such cases. If the site of the dural tear is known with sophisticated investigations such as CT myelography, then a blood patch is the treatment of choice. The outcome depends on the cause but in idiopathic cases, when the leak is presumed to be a dural tear or a nerve root avulsion, the symptoms usually settle spontaneously within several weeks (Lay 1997).

## Arterial dissection

Carotid dissection can occur either spontaneously or after minor injury to the neck (Mokri *et al.* 1986; Bogousslavsky *et al.* 1987; Fisher *et al.* 1987). The headache associated with carotid dissection is ipsilateral peri-orbital dull pain and can be associated with neck pain. The presence of a partial Horner's syndrome and in some cases retinal or cerebral transient ischaemic attack (TIA) may occur during the course of the condition. Patients presenting with peri-orbital headache and Horner's syndrome should alert the examining physician to the possibility. In many individuals dissection in the vertebral artery distribution can cause occipital headache and this can occur after neck injury and in some cases after neck manipulation (Mokri *et al.* 1988). Young individuals who present with recent-onset headache after such a history should always be investigated for this possibility. Carotid duplex Doppler sonography and MR angiography may reveal the abnormality but formal angiography is required, followed by anticoagulation in the form of heparin and warfarin. Recanalisation usually occurs in 6–8 weeks.

## Temporal arteritis

Generally speaking, temporal arteritis is rare and affects the elderly. Unilateral headache with temporal artery tenderness and a high ESR are classical presentations which should not be missed. The condition is a systemic vasculitis affecting middle-size arteries. There are general symptoms, including headache, fatigue, myalgia, jaw claudication and visual loss. The incidence increases with age and it is exceedingly rare in the under-50s. Association with polymyalgia rheumatica is seen in a third of patients. Weight loss, fever and even night sweats can occur. Although transient mono-ocular blindness can occur, the most feared complication is irreversible blindness, which can occur because of involvement of the ophthalmic artery.

Physical signs include induration and tenderness of the temporal or occipital scalp arteries on palpation and every effort should be made to start treatment with high-dose steroids early.

The problem here is that many of the elderly patients with this history have other problems, which makes the use of long-term steroids difficult. Associated illnesses make one hesitant in starting high-dose steroids, which should be maintained for a year or two in such individuals.

Performing a temporal artery biopsy in a general practice setting is perhaps impossible and referring such patients for urgent temporal artery biopsy is also difficult. The response to steroid treatment in the classical case is dramatic and if this happens, then the diagnosis is settled. Temporal artery biopsy should be performed early because using steroids, even for a few days, can lead to 'normalisation' of the biopsy. One is always taught that temporal arteritis can be present even with a low ESR or with a normal biopsy because of skip lesions.

## Trigeminal neuralgia

This condition in its classical form is easy to diagnose. The French term *tic douloureux* (painful spasm) is much more descriptive. The pain is severe, sharp and is within the trigeminal nerve distribution. It usually affects the second or third division but may involve the first division. The pain, as defined by the International Headache Society criteria, is paroxysmal lasting from few seconds to two minutes and is sudden, intense, sharp, superficial stabbing or burning in character. A classical history with trigger areas is vital for the diagnosis. Neurological examination is normal with no signs of trigeminal sensory involvement. Many individuals present with atypical facial pain, which is a completely different type of history and should not be confused with the classical sharp stabs of pain, which are triggered by certain movements or touching certain parts of the face, jaw or gum.

The majority of patients with trigeminal neuralgia, especially the elderly, have an aberrant vessel irritating the trigeminal nerve. Younger individuals may have demyelination as a cause or even neuromas and tumours irritating the trigeminal nerve. Investigating patients with trigeminal neuralgia is, therefore, indicated in the younger age group and in those who show abnormal signs on examining the trigeminal nerve territory. Patients with trigeminal neuralgia should have normal trigeminal sensation and normal motor function of the trigeminal nerve.

Treating trigeminal neuralgia is either medical with anti-convulsants such as carbamazepine, phenytoin and gabapentin, or using local injections of glycerol into the trigeminal ganglia. Over the last 20 years microvascular decompression through a posterior-fossa approach has been shown to be extremely successful in completely abolishing the pain and the need for drug therapy. This procedure is obviously invasive and is indicated in those patients who do not have any other medical problems and in those who have a reasonable life expectancy (Zakrzewska 1995). Stereotactic radiosurgery utilising the gamma ray knife is another method of treatment, which is non-invasive. This method has been applied to patients with trigeminal neuralgia in the last few years but long-term prognosis is not yet clear.

## Conclusion

This chapter has briefly reviewed some causes of headache and facial pain; taking a good history is the main method of differentiating sinister from more benign causes of headache.

### *References*

Adams HP, Kassell NF, Torner JC & Sahs AL (1983). CT and clinical correlation in recent aneurysmal subarachnoid haemorrhage: a prelimnary report of the cooperative aneurysm study. *Neurology* **33**, 981–8.

Arteriovenous Malformation Study Group (1999). Arteriovenous malformations in the brain in adults. *NEJM* **340**, 1812–18.

Bogousslavsky J, Despland PA & Regli F (1987). Spontaneous dissection with acute stroke. *Arch Neurol* **4**, 37–40.

Fisher CM, Ojemann RG & Robertson GH (1987). Spontaneous dissection of cervicocerebral arteries. *Can J Neurol Sci* **5**, 9–19.

Frishberg BM (1994). The utility of neuroimaging in the evaluation of headache in patients with normal neurologic examinations. *Neurology* **44**, 1191–7.

International Headache Society (1988). Classification and diagnostic criteria for headache disorders, cranial neuralgias, and facial pain. *Cephalalgia* **8**(Suppl.7), 1–96.

International Study of Unruptured Intracranial Aneurysms Investigators (1998). Unruptured intracranial aneurysm – risk of rupture and risk of surgical intervention. *N Engl J Med* **339**, 1725–33.

Lay CL, Campbell JK & Mokri B (1997). Low cerebrospinal fluid pressure headache. In *Blue books of practical neurology: headache* (ed. P Goadsby & SD Silberstein), pp.355–68. Butterworth-Heinemann, Boston.

Mokri B, Sundt TM, Houser OW & Piepgras DG (1986). Spontaneous dissection of the cervical internal carotid artery. *Ann Neurol* **19**, 126–38.

Mokri B, Houser W, Sandok BA & Piepgras DG (1988). Spontaneous dissections of the vertebral arteries. *Neurology* **38**, 880–5.

Quality Standards Subcommittee of the American Academy of Neurology (1994). Practice parameters: the utility of neuroimaging in the evaluation of headache in patients with normal neurologic examinations (Summary statement). *Neurology* **44**, 1353–4.

Ronkainen A, Hernesniemi J, Puranen M, Niemitukia L, Vanninen R, Ryynanen M, Kuivaniemi H & Tromp G (1997). Familial intracranial aneurysms. *Lancet* **349**, 380–4.

Zakrzewska JM (1995). Trigeminal neuralgia. In *Major problems in neurology*. WB Saunders, London, pp.157–70.

Chapter 3

# When to refer: a primary care perspective

*Manuela Fontebasso*

## Introduction
Migraine is a condition that has significant impact on quality of life (Liddell 1994), is extremely common (Lipton & Stewart 1994) and as such is ideally suited to management in a primary care setting. In trying to answer the question about when to refer it is important to understand why referral takes place. Referral may be within the primary health care team by or to any member of that team or on to secondary care for specialist advice.

## Understanding the needs of primary care
The pressure on GPs is ever increasing. Cost-effectiveness and efficiency are terms we have to contend with every day. As GPs we are constantly trying to balance patient demands and expectations with the ability of the system to respond.

The average migraine sufferer is female, aged 25–55 (Liddell 1994) and has 1–2 attacks per month. Only 30 per cent consult their GP, with the remainder using over-the-counter (OTC) medication to treat their symptoms. However, OTC medication will only abort 30–40 per cent of attacks, which leaves 60–70 per cent of sufferers suboptimally treated (MacGregor 1993).

## Why don't patients consult?
Patients seem to have a low expectation of treatment outcome; some are not aware of the new drugs launched over recent years and our deeper understanding of how best to use the drugs we have already. They do not realise that simple diet and lifestyle advice could have a dramatic effect on their condition.

Patients may have been to see their GPs in the past and found them dismissive of their symptoms. They may have found it difficult to explain the impact of their condition on their quality of life. Patients often complain that they have been given treatment that does not work but have never bothered to seek further advice. They see their GP as being a busy person and do not want to bother them with their headache.

## The GP perspective
GPs have many demands made upon their time. The average GP will have two surgeries a day, visits and possibly one other clinic. They are likely to see at least 170 patients per week (Emmanuel 1998). During the average 7–10-minute consultation, the GP

has to undertake a complex series of tasks as well as establish rapport with the patient. These tasks include:

- take a history
- examine the patient
- make a clinical diagnosis
- consider a broad treatment strategy
- explain the treatment to the patient
- explain the likely outcome
- explain the possible side-effects
- record the details of the consultation.

GPs are fortunate in their ability to use time. Taking a detailed headache and medication history takes time. Spending time at this stage with the patient may well prevent the need for referral later. If the GP can get the diagnosis right, then that will help to get the treatment right. One way of making this process less time-consuming is to give the patient a questionnaire to complete. The GP can arrange to review the questionnaires later, when a longer consultation is available.

The initial consultation is an opportunity to provide patients with information leaflets that will allow them to consider their symptoms in detail. Increasing their depth of knowledge will encourage them to develop a greater understanding of the options available to them. The second consultation will allow both the GP and the patient to consider the range of management options open to them. This direct involvement empowers the patient, will often result in improved treatment outcomes and should give them more realistic expectations.

## Management decisions

Having made the diagnosis of migraine, the GP and the patient have to decide what their needs and expectations are of the treatment options available (e.g. analgesics, analgesics at higher dose, soluble analgesics, anti-emetics, ergotamine, prophylaxis, oral triptans, triptans in non-oral form, complementary therapy).

Adopting a step-by-step approach will give the patient the greatest flexibility in identifying the best acute treatment strategy for them (Consumers' Association 1998). This will allow the introduction of prophylaxis at a threshold appropriate to the individual patient (Dowson *et al.* 1998). Involving the patient in the decision-making process will promote better outcomes and improve compliance. If the patient has a realistic expectation of treatment outcomes, then a more positive interaction between doctor and patient will result. Patients are more likely to return if the treatment is not effective or if they experience unacceptable side-effects.

GPs would benefit from guidance about when to consider prophylaxis, as this would improve management and reduce the need for referrals in the future. There needs to be a clear understanding of what prophylaxis offers to GPs and patients. Current Migraine in Primary Care Advisors (MIPCA) guidelines (Dowson *et al.* 1998) recommend a threshold of four or more migraine attacks per month for prophylaxis to be introduced. GPs and patients often have a low threshold for introducing prophylaxis as they expect all the attacks to be stopped. This is not the case. They perceive acute therapy options as being expensive but do not fully appreciate the cost of prophylactic medication.

Migraine sufferers do not want to take something on a daily basis unless it will dramatically reduce the number of attacks they experience and will cause them no side-effects: migraine has enough of a quality of life impact without taking medication which makes them feel worse.

The choice of drug will often depend on co-existing medical conditions. Once the choice has been made, it is important to start at a low dose to minimise the risk of side-effects. It is helpful to chart the frequency of attacks on a diary card to assess the response to the medication. The medication should be taken for a long enough period for it to have an impact (MIPCA guidelines suggest a period of three months). The patient should then be reviewed. If there has been no effect, the dose could be increased, repeating the process every three months until a response has been achieved or maximum dose has been reached or side-effects intervene.

Prophylaxis will only reduce the frequency of attacks by up to 50 per cent in up to 50 per cent of patients (Dowson *et al.* 1998). It is important that both the patient and the GP understand that effective acute treatment must be available for breakthrough attacks.

Decisions about treatment are complex (Dowson *et al.* 1998; Steiner *et al.* 1998). Several questions are to be considered, including:

- treatment history
- analgesic +/- anti-emetic or triptans
- which triptans?
- which dose?
- will there be side-effects?

The best place to start from is by taking an accurate medication history. This must include OTC as well as prescribed medication. It is imperative to clarify exactly what preparations, and at what dose, were used, and the timing of those doses.

There is no point in losing a patient's confidence by recommending something they have tried before and found ineffective. When planning future treatment strategies, it is important to evaluate past treatment, and the reasons for treatment failure need to be clarified.

Simple analgesia may not have worked for a number of reasons, including:

- it was too low a dose;
- it was taken too late in the attack;
- no anti-emetic was used;
- only oral medication was tried;
- different simple analgesics were not tried (e.g. aspirin, ibuprofen, indomethacin, naproxen, diclofenac, paracetamol).

Triptan therapy may have been ineffective because:

- it was taken in the aura phase;
- only oral preparations were used;
- it was taken too late;
- the patient did not have migraine.

Patients often stop using medication because:

- they experience side-effects;
- they have too high an expectation of effect;
- they only experience reduction in severity of headache and expect to be headache-free;
- they are concerned about the cost of treatment.

There are many questions that need answering. How can the GP meet patient need and not be overwhelmed by the time it would take to meet that need?

## Referral within the primary health care team

GPs can and do develop areas of special interest. In some practices it is possible to refer within the primary health care team for assessment of the patient who presents with headache. This is an effective use of skill-mix. The GP is then able to take a full history, examine the patient and, after making the diagnosis, be in a position to discuss a treatment strategy with the patient.

It is at this point that many GPs would refer on to the practice nurse. With training and a sound knowledge base, nurses are ideally placed to negotiate with the patient many of the diet and lifestyle changes essential for effective headache and migraine management. They have many opportunities to identify patients who suffer from migraine during the course of their routine work. They may refer on to the GP for more formal diagnosis.

Community pharmacists are also ideally placed to identify patients who are abusing analgesic medication. They can offer advice to patients who present to them complaining of headache. By making suggestions about what is the most appropriate medication to take, they can reduce the risk of headache caused by medication misuse developing in the future. They may also refer to other members of the primary health care team.

Health visitors, in their role with the under-5s, are in regular opportunistic contact with young women who are most likely to suffer from headache.

Developing a practice protocol for headache management would enable all members of the primary health care team to make the most effective use of the skill-mix available within the practice.

## Referrals to a specialist clinic

There are many reasons why patients get referred to a specialist clinic, including: diagnostic difficulties, patients refractory to treatment and patient demand. During the course of my employment at the headache clinic in York, I have always found the general quality of referrals to be of a high standard. It is not always easy to make the diagnosis of migraine. The IHS guidelines (Headache Classification Committee of the International Headache Society 1988) do offer some assistance but it is still only a framework. Migraine does not always neatly fit into the slots available. It is helpful to make the correct diagnosis, as this will usually guide you to the appropriate treatment option. Difficulties in making the diagnosis are usually due to the presence of more than one type of headache. Onward referral at this point may well be the most appropriate course of action.

Patients refractory to treatment may well be at a stalemate because a step-by-step approach has not been used. Some of the reasons for treatment failure have already been discussed. Onward referral at this point may be the most appropriate course of action so that a fresh start can be made.

Patients are increasingly being made aware of their rights. They do increasingly and sometimes rightly demand referral to a specialist centre. They may feel that their GP has been dismissive of their symptoms. They may feel that they continue to experience a significant impact on quality of life despite the treatment prescribed or suggested. Weekly magazines, newspapers and television are all responsible for raising the profile of health issues. There is increasing awareness of what options are available and patients demand referral so that they can access that advice and information. There is little to be gained by refusing referral at this point.

Developing a practice protocol for the management of headache and migraine would encourage the most cost-effective use of referrals. The majority of patients would be managed in the primary care setting and only those causing management or diagnostic difficulties or who might have sinister underlying pathology would be referred.

A step-by-step approach to treatment would suggest the use of simple analgesia and if this is not effective in controlling migraine symptoms then the use of a triptan would be appropriate (Dowson *et al.* 1998; Steiner *et al.* 1998). Triptans are, rightly or wrongly, perceived as expensive, but they can be extremely effective in aborting the acute migraine attack, and a patient who finds an effective acute treatment is usually delighted. They might only then request referral or further assessment if the frequency of attacks continues to have a significant impact on quality of life. Using a triptan is much cheaper than an unnecessary referral and often a cheaper option to short-, medium- or even long-term prophylaxis.

Patients do not need to be on prophylaxis long term. The use of prophylaxis needs to be regularly reviewed to ensure that treatment is reducing attack frequency (Steiner *et al.* 1998). If it does, then it should be discontinued after 3–6 months. Patients need to have a realistic expectation of what prophylaxis can offer them. It needs to be taken for long enough at the right dose to be effective. It will not stop all their attacks so they will still need effective rescue medication for breakthrough attacks.

Daily headache is not migraine. There is increasing recognition of the diagnostic and management problems associated with chronic daily headache and medication misuse headache (Dowson *et al.* 1998; Steiner *et al.* 1998). Patients who present with more than one type of headache will often require a specialist package of care. It is important to ask the question: do you have more than one type of headache?

## What will help primary care?

A common set of management goals within the primary health care team would offer consistency in the approach given to patients (Dowson *et al.* 1998). Guidelines generated between primary and secondary care would enable all members of the primary health care team to have access to management solutions that could improve treatment outcomes. A structured approach about when to refer would ensure the most cost-effective use of resources.

The goals listed in Box 3.1 have been developed by MIPCA and are valid in the primary and secondary care setting. Patients can identify with them. By working together as a team, primary and secondary care professionals can ensure that patients can regain control of their headache symptoms.

GPs will be encouraged to use a step-by step approach to treat the acute attack. Prophylaxis will be introduced at a threshold relevant to the individual patient. Referral could be made when one or more triptans have been tried. It may be that initial treatment has not been effective. It may be that the treatment has been effective but the frequency of attacks requires a specialist package of care.

## Serious causes of headache

As GPs we are all concerned about missing sinister pathology. Headache is the most common presenting symptom and may form up to 40 per cent of all consultations (Patten 1996). The majority of patients who present with headache are worried that they have a brain tumour. Cancer is a word that generates fear in doctor and patient

---

**Box 3.1** Goals of migraine management

- To understand the impact of migraine
- To allow patients to manage their migraine without disruption to their day-to-day activities, work, social and family life
- To establish the most effective treatment regimen
- To ensure that treatment allows the patient to resume normal activities as quickly as possible
- Where possible, to identify what triggers the patient's attacks

**Box 3.2** Serious causes of headache

- Intracranial tumours
- Meningitis
- Subarachnoid haemorrhage
- Temporal arteritis

alike. Patients who experience their first aura are often convinced they are having a stroke. However, sinister pathology (see Box 3.2) will occur in less than 2 per cent of all headaches. The most important tool that the GP has is in taking the history and examining the patient. There will always be something in the history or the examination that will raise the index of suspicion that further investigation is required. As GPs we know our patients, and intuition will often play a significant part in the assessment process and should not be ignored. Spending time with patients, explaining and educating them may be all that they require.

Specific features in the patient's history or examination usually suggest sinister pathology. Intracranial tumours are likely to present with focal neurological signs or symptoms. A person suffering from meningitis is obviously ill. An individual with a subarachnoid haemorrhage may or may not have clear-cut symptoms and signs: admission and investigation may be the only way of making the diagnosis. This is particularly true in the elderly where a low threshold of suspicion is often needed (Steiner *et al.* 1998). Headache is a constant feature of temporal arteritis. Accurate diagnosis is needed to ensure that appropriate treatment is initiated. The erythrocyte sedimentation rate is not always useful because it can be normal and it may be raised in the elderly in the presence of other pathology. Examination can be helpful but not always reliable. Temporal artery biopsy is often necessary to make an accurate diagnosis. Treatment is with steroids at high dose and may be long term so the diagnosis must be correct (Steiner *et al.* 1998).

Other causes of headache that may pose problems include:

- carbon monoxide poisoning
- post-traumatic headache
- idiopathic intracranial hypertension.

Carbon monoxide poisoning is an uncommon but potentially fatal cause of headache. In 1996/7 21 people died in the UK, with a further 90 people experiencing ill health from carbon monoxide poisoning (Steiner *et al.* 1998).

## When to refer?

As GPs it can be difficult to decide when to refer a patient. There are times when intuition takes over and that should not be ignored. There are times when following a set of guidelines pays dividends (see Box 3.3).

**Box 3.3** When to refer?

- First worst headache, especially over 50
- Clinically significant physical signs
- Recently changed headache
- Out-of-character headache
- More than one type of headache
- Refractory to treatment
- Patient demand
- Children and adoloscents

If a patient experiences their first worst-ever headache, then careful assessment is needed. It may suggest sinister pathology especially if they are over the age of 50. I can remember one patient seen at the headache clinic in York who presented with what sounded like migraine without aura. He was 52 years old with no previous history of headache. An MR angiography showed a large arteriovenous malformation that required surgical intervention.

Clinically significant physical signs will require referral and investigation. If the nature, type or character of the headache have changed, then investigation is often justified, because there may be a change in the underlying pathology.

As GPs we know our patients. We know those who are always at the surgery and we know those who rarely visit us. If a patient comes with a headache that is out of character, then it needs to be taken seriously. Intuition has a part to play.

A patient suffering from more than one type of headache, especially if the second headache is due to medication misuse, would benefit from referral. These patients often require a special package of care best undertaken in the secondary care setting. Some require hospital admission for drug withdrawal (Dowson *et al.* 1998; Steiner *et al.* 1998).

Patients failing to respond to acute or prophylactic therapy will often benefit from specialist input: it gives them a fresh perspective and encourages them to take responsibility for their own treatment.

Patients usually demand referral to a specialist headache clinic because they appreciate the variety of knowledge and skills that they can access. Counsellors, nurses and physiotherapists do offer broad management strategies. Patients are often hungry for information and welcome the opportunity to speak to people who understand their problems.

Children and adolescents are a difficult group to treat. They can respond well to simple analgesics and experience a significant placebo effect when tried on triptans. Assessment at a specialist centre will often facilitate the management process and reassure parents that there is no sinister pathology.

## Effective referral

Raising awareness about the different types of headache will improve understanding of the diagnostic dilemmas and encourage effective use of the skills of primary and secondary care professionals.

Educating all members of the primary health care team will do much to getting the diagnosis right. The right diagnosis will in turn promote the adoption of the right treatment strategies.

Patients and doctors both need to have realistic expectations of acute and prophylactic treatment. This will promote better treatment outcomes and reduce the need for specialist referral.

Migraine is not just a headache. It has a significant quality of life impact and deserves to be treated proactively and effectively. Treating migraine proactively is very rewarding: when you get it right, the patient is extremely grateful. It does take time but it is time well spent.

Always remember, when writing your referral letter, to write down in detail the medication history. This should include:

- names and doses of all drugs tried
- how long each drug was used at that dose
- what drugs produced side-effects
- OTC medication.

Patients can rarely remember what tablets they are taking now, let alone remember what had been tried over the past year. The hospital specialist does not want to lose the confidence of the patient by trying something that has already been used in the past, at the right dose, for long enough and did not work.

## Conclusion

Headache is a very common presenting symptom. Migraine is a very common condition. They are ideally suited to proactive management in the primary care setting.

Referrals can be made within the primary health care team to offer patients a step-by-step approach to treatment. Working to a common protocol would facilitate this process.

Referral to secondary care would be made once first-stage interventions had been tried or the history or examination of the patient suggested more sinister pathology.

## *References*

Consumers' Association (1998). Managing migraine. *Drugs and Therapeutics Bulletin* **36**(6), 41–4.
Dowson A J, Gruffydd-Jones K, Hackett G *et al.* (1998). *Migraine: key facts.* Essential information from MIPCA (Migraine in Primary Care Advisors).
Emmanuel E (1998). GPs are the primary consultants. *BMA New Review* Nov, 36.

Headache Classification Committee of the International Headache Society (1988). Classification and diagnostic criteria for headache disorders, cranial neuralgias and facial pain. *Cephalalgia* **8**(Suppl.7), 1–96.

Liddell J (1994). Migraine: the patient's perspective. *Rev Contemp Pharmacother* **5**, 253–7.

Lipton R B & Stewart W F (1994). The epidemiology of migraine. *Eur Neurol* **34** (Suppl.2), 6–11.

MacGregor E A (1993). Prescribing for migraine. *Prescriber* **33**(2), 50–8.

Patten J (1996). *Neurological differential diagnosis* 2nd edn, Springer, pp. 357–71.

Steiner TJ, MacGregor EA & Davies PTG (1998). *BASH guidelines for all doctors in the diagnosis and management of migraine*. British Association for the Study of Headache.

Chapter 4

# When to refer: a secondary care perspective

*Richard Peatfield*

## Introduction

A wide variety of diseases have headache among their primary symptoms, and many more will also cause headache, although the physician's attention is then usually more appropriately directed to other symptoms which are likely to be more diagnostically significant. A reasonable list of the most likely causes of headache in patients seeking medical attention would include: migraine; tension headache; cluster headache (migrainous neuralgia); cervical spondylosis; temporal arteritis; sinusitis; trigeminal neuralgia; atypical facial pain; subarachnoid haemorrhage; meningitis and causes of raised intracranial pressure such as tumours, abscesses and benign intracranial hypertension.

The relative frequency of these causes is dependent on the circumstances in which the series of patients has been collected. Migraine and cluster headache are overwhelmingly the most frequent diagnoses in patients attending a migraine clinic, whereas the majority of patients with headache attending a general neurology clinic in a district hospital have tension-type headache. In series from Accident & Emergency departments (see, for example, Fodden *et al.* 1989), in which many of the patients will be complaining of 'the worst headache of my life', structural causes are substantially more frequent, though still only perhaps 10–20 per cent of total numbers. Under these circumstances it is particularly important to consider subarachnoid haemorrhage, meningitis and the causes of raised intracranial pressure. This chapter, in contrast, is more concerned with patients consulting their general practitioner (GP) with long-standing headache, either constant or episodic, and the factors which should lead the GP to seek further advice about the patient's management.

## The GP's role in initiating referral

In the Princess Margaret Migraine Clinic at Charing Cross Hospital, London, a significant proportion of the patients have referred themselves. They usually contact a migraine charity or patient association in the first instance, and are very properly told to ask their GP to write a referral letter. It is only right that hospital specialists should accept that, however benign these headaches may be, many do require the assistance of a specialist clinic before a patient's anxieties are allayed. Some, of course, can be reassured at a single GP consultation, but others should be referred for a specialist opinion, which can often be completed on a single visit.

Perhaps half the referrals at the Princess Margaret Migraine Clinic are initiated by the GP. The reasons for referral vary and are considered below.

## The diagnosis is clear but hospital management is required

In many cases the diagnosis is straightforward but hospital technology is necessary for appropriate management. A number of diagnoses fall into this category, including subarachnoid haemorrhage and other headache of sudden onset in which full hospital-based investigation is required to exclude a subarachnoid haemorrhage (it is now well established that this cannot be done on clinical grounds alone and all these patients require a CT brain scan and a lumbar puncture before the diagnostic label of 'thunderclap headache' can be applied (Harling *et al.* 1989)). Clearly, any patients in whom ventricular blood or even an aneurysm is demonstrated on the CT brain scan should be referred directly to a neurosurgeon. However, up to one-third of patients experiencing a subarachnoid haemorrhage will have a normal CT brain scan, and in these circumstances examination of the cerebrospinal fluid (CSF) is essential. In one series about one-third of patients with thunderclap headache had subsequent more convincing migraine attacks (many of these had a long history of such attacks), about one-third had cervical spondylosis, and the remaining third were best labelled 'psychogenic' (Wijdicks *et al.* 1988; Harling *et al.* 1989).

Patients with meningitis also fall into this category and again require full investigation, usually after antibiotic treatment has been initiated.

Any patients with focal neurological signs, during or particularly between their attacks of headache, should also be investigated as a matter of urgency – a substantial minority of these will have structural abnormalities in the brain causing the headache, and many of the rest will have small infarcts, which may justify further investigation themselves, though the neurologist may conclude that the infarct is part of the migrainous process. Patients with papilloedema also fall into the category, as do patients with headache induced by (and not merely worsened by) coughing and headache caused or relieved by repositioning of the patient's head, which is occasionally due to an intraventricular tumour, such as a colloid cyst.

## Progressive history without signs necessitating a scan

This is, perhaps, the commonest single reason for GP-initiated referrals. Many of these are entirely appropriate. It has to be accepted that a very small proportion of such patients do actually have causative structural abnormalities. In a series of 725 patients seen in the Princess Margaret Migraine Clinic between 1979 and 1981, for example, there were two such patients, one with a subdural haematoma and one with a pituitary tumour. At the same time, there were two patients with temporal arteritis, two with sinusitis and six with cervical spondylosis, with a vast majority of the remainder having migraine, tension-type headache or cluster headache. It will, of course, be appreciated that the patients with temporal arteritis would have had a negative CT scan and the diagnosis would have been missed had this been performed without appropriate preliminary clinical assessment.

There is now an extensive literature on the likelihood of finding a relevant structural lesion when scanning patients of this kind. Honig & Charney (1982), for example, performed a retrospective study of 72 children with headache due to brain tumour between 1965 and 1978 – a series that was, therefore, started before the introduction of the CT brain scan. They found that 68 of these patients (94 per cent) had abnormal signs at the time of diagnosis and these abnormalities developed in 85 per cent of the patients within two months of the onset of their headache. Honig & Charney concluded that attention to abnormal features or signs would have led to the diagnosis in 96 per cent of their patients within four months of onset.

The study of Mitchell *et al.* (1993) approached this problem from the opposite direction. They assembled a series of 350 patients, whose mean age was 33, with a chief complaint of headache, regardless of the presence or absence of physical signs. Only seven of these had clinically significant CT scan findings, and all seven had an abnormal physical or neurological examination, or unusual clinical symptomatology. Three of these patients had had headache for less than a week and five for less than four weeks. Only one patient, with a falx meningioma, had had headache for three months, and in the remaining patient the duration of the headache was uncertain. Mitchell *et al.* concluded that 'routine brain CT scanning of headache patients with a normal general and neurological examination, and no unusual clinical symptomatology, is a low-yield study'. In the series assembled by Weingarten *et al.* (1992) there were no significant abnormalities in 89 scans performed for chronic isolated headache without physical signs, even when these patients were followed up for up to two years. They also studied 40 other patients with malignant brain tumour, recording that none had chronic isolated headache at the time of diagnosis and only two had sought medical attention with isolated headache, but they developed physical signs by the time of diagnosis. Weingarten *et al.* concluded that less than one patient in 10,000 without physical signs has a tumour. They excluded a number of patients using the criteria listed in Box 4.1; these criteria would form a reasonable checklist for performing a scan in a specialist outpatient context.

Similar conclusions were drawn from the large series assembled by Dumas *et al.* (1994). They had 373 patients with a history of headache for over six months, without epilepsy or physical signs, which constituted about 10 per cent of their outpatient population in their neurology clinic. Of these patients, 287 were scanned because of the increasing severity of their symptoms or resistance to treatment, and 78 because of a change in the pattern of their headaches. Eight further patients were only scanned because of a family history of a structural lesion. Dumas *et al.* performed a total of 402 scans finding minor structural abnormalities in 14 and significant findings only in four – these were two osteomas, one low-grade glioma and one aneurysm. At that time, an unenhanced CT brain scan cost $83 in their

**Box 4.1** Criteria for investigating a patient with headache

Neurological symptoms
Abnormal neurological signs
Persistent visual symptoms, or blurred vision
Personality change, cognitive deficit, or memory loss
Head injury less than 4 months before
Known cancer
Known or suspected HIV infection
Seizures
History of subarachnoid or intracranial bleeding
Prior neurosurgical procedure

*Source:* Weingarten *et al.* (1992)

establishment and an enhanced scan $204; they calculated that the cost per treatable lesion exceeded $18,000.

My colleague, Dr Fayyez Ahmed, performed an audit of scans undertaken in the Princess Margaret Migraine Clinic in 1994. In that year we saw 1,725 patients of whom 1,108 were new. We did a total of 46 scans, 38 on new patients and 8 on follow-up patients. The reasons that Dr Ahmed assigned for these scans are listed in Table 4.1. Of the 14 patients with atypical headache, there were only two abnormalities, and these were both lacunar vascular abnormalities of uncertain significance. Fourteen patients, all with physical signs, were scanned because of suspected pathology, and in only three there were significant findings: there was one cerebral tumour, one orbital pseudo-tumour and one patient with benign intracranial hypertension. Dr Ahmed acknowledges that many of these scans are necessary to maintain the confidence of the patients, but the yield is extremely low.

In the vast majority of patients with cerebral tumours the tumour comes to light either because of seizures or because of focal brain dysfunction (such as hemiparesis, visual field defects, sensory symptoms or signs, dysphasia or personality change, or because of papilloedema). While it is very rare for patients with cerebral tumours to present with headache alone, most will develop headache as the pathology advances.

**Table 4.1** Audit of Princess Margaret Migraine Clinic patients seen in 1994 (n=1,725)

46 scans (38 on new patients, 8 on follow-ups)
No. of scans:

| | | |
|---|---|---|
| 10 | Reassurance | All negative |
| 8 | 'As a last resort' | All negative |
| 14 | Atypical or late onset | 2: lacunes |
| 14 | Suspected pathology | 3 (all 3 with signs): cerebral tumour, benign intracranial hypertension, orbital pseudo-tumour |

**Box 4.2** Hazards of unnecessary scanning

*False negatives*
Temporal arteritis
Small subarachnoid haemorrhage
Arnold-Chiari malformations
Cervical spondylosis

*False positives*
UBOs/infarcts
Irrelevant meningiomas etc.

*Undue emphasis on diagnosis rather than management*

The hazards of unnecessary scanning have to be appreciated (Box 4.2). The dangers of offering reassurance on the basis of a normal scan without proper clinical assessment cannot be overemphasised and, in addition, most neurologists will recall spending some time explaining the lack of significance of some relatively trivial abnormality to an anxious patient investigated by a colleague.

## Difficult management problems

There are a number of patients whose headaches prove intractable and who are likely to benefit from more specialist care. Common examples are temporal arteritis, which often requires a biopsy of the temporal artery, and certainly requires serial measurements of the ESR, often for several years. Most general practitioners have a relatively limited experience of cluster headache, which is an extremely severe pain that often proves intractable to several lines of management, and it can realistically be argued that all such patients should be under the care of a neurologist.

Many of the referrals to the Princess Margaret Migraine Clinic state, usually by implication, that the patient is proving something of a budgetary embarrassment because of the large quantities of triptan drugs they are taking. While some of these patients may respond to cheaper alternatives such as anti-inflammatory agents combined with an anti-emetic, others may benefit from regular prophylactic treatment and one of the many roles of a migraine clinic is to offer this when appropriate. The use of a second dose of triptan to treat a recurrent headache is common, but there are a number of patients who give themselves doses on several consecutive days, and these may benefit from either stopping the treatment completely or by using a longer-acting triptan with a lower recurrence rate.

Other patients prove unresponsive to several orthodox lines of management. There is a substantial list of second-line agents, both analgesic and prophylactic, which may be suitable for migraine patients and many referrals to the Princess

Margaret Migraine Clinic benefit from these. Other causes of intractable headache, such as analgesic abuse, usually of codeine, but occasionally of ergotamine, and simultaneous depression are covered in Chapters 5 and 6 of this book. In many other cases, the GP has been a little reluctant to use a dose of medication large enough to influence the patient's headache and neurologists find themselves either using the same drugs at doses two or three times higher or trying to exploit the admittedly subtle differences between the triptan preparations now available.

## Genuine diagnostic difficulties

Few patients attending a migraine clinic provide much of a diagnostic problem, but it is worth singling out the following:

- New headache in older people is uncommon – most of these patients will admit to a long past history of migraine and in some others there is a recent change in hormonal treatment which can account for the change in headache pattern. Trigeminal neuralgia is unusual and easily identifiable by appropriate questioning. Although temporal arteritis is potentially the most serious diagnosis, cervical spondylosis is by far the commonest cause of *new* headache in the elderly. Although most of these patients have occipital pain in the mid-line radiating only as far as the vertex, in others it seems to reach the forehead, perhaps because of the overlap between descending trigeminal pathways and ascending cervical pathways in the brainstem. It is always prudent to check the ESR as occasional patients have simultaneous temporal arteritis, but the majority of these improve with a small dose of a long-acting non-steroidal agent such as diclofenac.
- New headache in younger patients is usually still due to migraine, though this overlaps with the tension-type headache. Many patients with a previous history of episodic migraine come to neurological attention because their headache 'transforms' into a more chronic form. Anyone seeing such patients, whether in general practice or later, should consider either analgesic abuse, or the administration of oestrogens, or depression as possible causes, as appropriate advice may well settle the headache with few, if any, investigations.

## Conclusions

In conclusion, a neurologist practising in a headache clinic spends his or her time:

- reassuring the worried
- investigating a few
- starting migraine prophylaxis when this can be justified
- improving acute treatment.

## References

Dumas MD, Pexman JHW & Kreeft JH (1994). Computed tomography evaluation of patients with chronic headache. *Canad Med Assoc J* **151**, 1447–52.

Fodden DI, Peatfield RC & Milsom PL (1989). Beware the patient with a headache in the accident and emergency department. *Archives of Emergency Medicine* **6**, 7–12.

Harling DW, Peatfield RC, Van Hille PT & Abbott RJ (1989). Thunderclap headache: is it migraine? *Cephalalgia* **9**, 87–90.

Honig PJ & Charney EB (1982). Children with brain tumor headaches. Distinguishing features. *Am J Dis Child* **136**, 121–4.

Mitchell CS, Osborn RE & Grosskreutz SR (1993) Computed tomography in the headache patient: is routine evaluation really necessary? *Headache* **33**, 82–6.

Weingarten S, Kleinman M, Elperin L & Larson EB (1992). The effectiveness of cerebral imaging in the diagnosis of chronic headache. *Arch Int Med* **152**, 2457–62.

Wijdicks EFM, Kerkhoff H & Van Gijn J (1988). Long term follow-up of 71 patients with thunderclap headache mimicking subarachnoid haemorrhage. *Lancet* **2**, 68–70.

Chapter 5

# Psychiatric perspectives on headache

*Geir Madland and Charlotte Feinmann*

## Introduction

Many aspects of headache remain poorly understood. The lifetime incidence of headache is nearly 100 per cent, yet only a small percentage of sufferers actively seek treatment from health services.

What prompts individuals to seek treatment? Is there a gender bias, and are cultural factors involved? Diagnosis of a particular class of headache is then made on the basis of self-report of subjective symptoms and elicitation of signs through apparently objective testing. How reliable are these criteria? Subsequent referral to a neurologist is followed by a lengthy spell on a waiting list. What effect might this delay have on the individual? What is the patient to make of progressively complex medical tests, are they necessary, and is the neurologist best equipped to help? With reference to aetiology, is migraine determined by personality traits and is there a shared biological origin with depression? As headaches continue, how is the individual affected by this persisting condition? Does one's way of thinking change with time, and do cognitions, such as illness perceptions, contribute to the maintenance of symptoms? What is the relationship with stress? What needs to happen for treatment to succeed and how should outcome be assessed? What are the dangers of chronic self-medication?

These questions are addressed below, and recommendations are made for future clinical management and research.

## Seeking treatment

The lifetime incidence of headache is probably close to 100 per cent (Ho *et al.* 1997) and nearly three-quarters of the population report recent head pain (see, for example, Koutantji *et al.* 1998). Using International Headache Society criteria, the prevalence of headache over 12 months in the general adult population is approximately 10 per cent for migraine and 20–30 per cent for frequent (more than monthly) tension-type headache (Rasmussen & Olesen 1994), yet only one half of migraine sufferers, and less than one-sixth of tension-type headache sufferers, seek medical advice (Rasmussen *et al.* 1992).

*What prompts individuals to seek treatment, and how do they differ from those who don't?*

Frequency and severity of symptoms are likely to be the chief factors in determining treatment-seeking but these variables are evidently subjective and, hence, psychological factors may well be influential. Clinic patients report greater occupational disability than do headache sufferers not seeking treatment, even after controlling for headache severity (Ziegler & Paolo 1996).

*Is there a gender bias, and are cultural influences involved?*

There is a female preponderance in both migraine and tension-type headache, with male-to-female ratios of approximately 1:2.5 and 1:1.5 respectively, in the general population (Rasmussen & Olesen 1994). These gender differences may be due to hormonal or psychological influences but, in any event, are compounded by the greater use of health services by women. Ethnic and cultural differences also affect pain report: for example, Americans of European descent report less post-operative dental pain than do those of Black American or Latino descent (Faucett *et al.* 1994). Migraine has, in the past, been considered an illness of the professional classes, and this may reflect a barrier to consultation in low-income groups (Lipton *et al.* 1992).

## Being diagnosed

Diagnosis of a particular class of headache is made on the basis of self-report of subjective symptoms and elicitation of signs through apparently objective testing.

*How reliable are these criteria?*

There is good evidence for a fundamental distinction between migraine and tension-type headache (Rasmussen & Olesen 1994). The former appears to be the manifestation of a basic neurochemical disorder, while the latter has distinct relations with stress. The occurrence of tension-type headache in migraine sufferers should not, therefore, present any conceptual problem (Ulrich *et al.* 1996). However, psychophysiological tests, including frontal electromyography (EMG) and temporal blood volume pulse (BVP), temporal and finger skin temperature, fail to differentiate between the two disorders (Lichstein *et al.* 1991) and the diagnosis is made on the history.

## Becoming a specialist's case

Referral by a general practitioner to a neurologist may be followed by a lengthy spell on a waiting list, as a result of budgetary constraints and the relative lack of urgency.

*What effect might this delay have on the individual?*

Specialist pain clinic populations exhibit greater prevalence of psychiatric morbidity than do population-based or primary care samples (von Korff & Simon 1996).

This suggests either that it is only those individuals who find it difficult to adjust to their pain, and are consequently distressed, who end up in specialist clinics; or that individuals become distressed over the time it takes to get them there. The lack of prospective studies of chronic pain precludes any conclusions.

*What is the patient to make of progressively complex medical tests?*
*Are they necessary, and is the neurologist best equipped to help?*

The problem with exhaustive testing such as EMG, vascular studies and imaging, is the re-inforcement of the medical model of illness. With each negative test, the patient may well become convinced of the existence of an undetected organic lesion. It has recently been suggested that 'greater and earlier exposure to the primary health care setting would modify doctors' beliefs about the appropriateness of extensive physical investigation, and the relative values of clinical histories and physical examination findings' (Peveler 1998, p.95). A neuroimaging examination is only indicated with an atypical clinical picture, which is rare (Jelencsik 1998). Neurologists may view pain relief as the most important aim of management and thus fail to provide adequate explanation and reassurance (Edmeads 1998). Yet premature reassurance by itself may actually prove harmful in attempting, via verbal and non-verbal cues, to persuade the patient of the absence of disease (Coia & Morley 1998). In any event, a busy neurology outpatient clinic does not lend itself to patient listening to what may be a lengthy and complex history, nor to advice and counselling thereon.

Ideally, a multidisciplinary team should undertake the management of headache patients, but this may not be financially practical. Certainly, the liaison psychiatrist has much to contribute in the elicitation and interpretation of a pain history, and in the informed and informative provision of antidepressant medication as an aid to management.

## Being a migraine sufferer

*Is migraine determined by personality traits?*

There is no evidence for a typical migraine personality (Kohler & Kosanic 1992). Migraine sufferers do, however, exhibit greater neuroticism than controls (Leijdekkers & Passchier 1990; Breslau *et al.* 1996; Persson 1997). Yet, the concept of the neurotic personality might be better considered as a tendency to perceive greater stress than others, and again, in the absence of prospective studies, one cannot determine whether this tendency derives from the experience of migraine or vice versa.

There may well be a role for previous experience of pain and distress in predisposing adults to symptoms. A significant positive relationship has been shown between depression and a history of childhood sexual and physical abuse in patients with chronic pain (Goldberg 1994). The familial occurrence of headaches is likely to be encouraged by modelling, especially in the absence of any evidence for a genetic basis (Bahra & Goadsby 1998).

*Is there a shared biological origin with depression?*

The risk of developing depression in migraine sufferers, relative to population controls, is virtually identical to the risk for developing migraine in depressives (3.2 and 3.1 respectively, Breslau *et al.* 1994). Together with evidence of comorbidity from familial and biochemical studies and the therapeutic efficacy of antidepressant agents in migraine, this association has led to the postulation of a common pathophysiological mechanism for migraine and depression (Bahra & Goadsby 1998). The increased risk of major depression in migraine sufferers strengthens the need for psychiatric liaison but does not support the psychodynamic notion of migraine as masked depression (Blumer & Heilbronn 1982).

## Thinking as a chronic patient

*How is the individual affected by this persisting condition?*

Tension-type headache sufferers show mildly more anxious and depressed moods (Hatch *et al.* 1991), much greater fear of severe pain (Hursey & Jacks 1992), and more frequent suppression of anger (Hatch *et al.* 1991), than do controls.

Chronic daily headache, considered to be transformed migraine in many cases, is associated with high anxiety levels (Mongini *et al.* 1997); while migraine is associated with depression (Verri *et al.* 1998). Rates of suicidal ideation and suicide attempts are increased in migraine with aura, especially with coexisting depression (Breslau 1992).

Quality of life studies have demonstrated the impact of recurrent headaches. The burden of migraine may be equal to, or worse than, that of arthritis, diabetes or low back pain (Solomon 1997). It would appear to be the emotional component of the pain that predicts a fall in health-related quality of life, rather than headache diagnosis, frequency or severity (Passchier *et al.* 1996).

*Does one's way of thinking change with time?*

Although there is no evidence of associated cognitive impairment *per se* (Leijdekkers *et al.* 1990), Demjen *et al.* (1990, p.427) have described a cognitive shift with headache of increasing severity 'whereby the patient's primary concern moves from situational and interpersonal distress to distress associated with the disorder itself'. They stress the impact of both symptom intensity and duration in increasing headache-related distressing thoughts and feelings.

*Do cognitions, such as illness perceptions, contribute to the maintenance of symptoms?*

Other chronic conditions show a relationship between illness perceptions, disability and mood. Chronic fatigue syndrome patients, who consider their condition to be serious and beyond control or cure, report greater physical, social and mental health

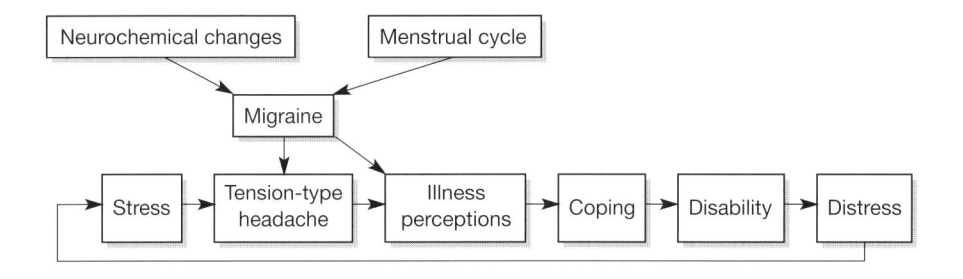

**Figure 5.1** A scheme to illustrate the hypothesised relations between psychological factors in headache

impairment (Heijmans 1998). Similar relationships may exist in chronic headache patients but have not been investigated.

The perception of stress is an important factor in symptom recurrence, certainly in tension-type headache (De Benedettis & Lorenzetti 1992). Both life events and daily 'hassles' have been studied, and it would appear that, while life events may trigger hassles, it is the perceived severity of those hassles that best predicts headache frequency and intensity (Fernandez & Sheffield 1996). Physiological disregulation of stress response may be involved in tension-type headache but not in migraine (Davis *et al.* 1998), although migraine sufferers show increased cardiovascular activity in response to stress compared with controls (Stronks *et al.* 1998). Tension-type headache sufferers may fail to pay adequate attention to environmental information when appraising stressful events; while migraine may be associated with delayed recovery of cardiovascular response to stress (Holm *et al.* 1997). It may be the way in which headache sufferers respond to stressful events that determines the onset and intensity of attacks (Marlowe 1998).

There is likely to be a complex temporal relationship between stress, mood and migraine (Spierings *et al.* 1997). In coping tests, migraine patients appear to be more negative as to their anticipated future activities than do cluster headache patients (Blomkvist *et al.* 1997). In female migraine sufferers, headache is associated with stress during the premenstrual and ovulatory phases. This supports a relationship between the menstrual cycle, the stress-appraisal-coping process, and migraine (Holm *et al.* 1996). Figure 5.1 shows a putative scheme.

## Breaking the cycle

### *What needs to happen for treatment to succeed?*

Successful treatment of headaches is associated with reduction in disability, improvement in quality of life, amelioration of mood, positive adaptation of coping strategies in response to stress, and enhanced perceived control over pain. These are not all to be achieved with a simple pill. For a drug to be effective in reducing the pain of headaches, its prescription must be accompanied by expectation of its efficacy. Consequently, should that efficacy fail to meet expectation, the pain may become less responsive at the next attempt.

The doctor-patient interaction plays an important role in nurturing expectation but subtle cognitive and conditioned responses are also likely to be involved (Wall 1994). Placebo response is greatly enhanced by the experience of effective analgesia (Voudouris *et al.* 1990) and, hence, an individual's belief in the efficacy of any therapy is greatly enhanced if it appears to improve any aspect of the pain, even if that improvement cannot ultimately be attributed to the therapy itself but may in fact be a spontaneous remission. This may account for some of the effectiveness of antidepressant agents in chronically recurrent pain, including headache. Even in an apparently non-depressed pain patient such agents can be expected to affect mood, which is an aspect of the pain experience, thus breaking the cycle of stress, pain, disability and distress. Pain is adversive, and depression may be the result of adversity, so the finding of a shared neurochemistry involving serotonin is not altogether surprising.

Tricyclic antidepressants, notably amitriptyline, have been established to be of benefit, at least in the short term, in reducing the duration of daily tension-type headaches, while having less effect on more episodic complaints (Gobel *et al.* 1994; Cerbo *et al.* 1998). However, when strict criteria for improvement in duration, frequency and intensity are employed, the effect of amitriptyline is no greater than placebo (Pfaffenrath *et al.* 1993). In addition, despite the difficulties in comparing such disparate treatment modalities, cognitive behavioural therapy has been shown to be slightly more effective than amitriptyline (Holroyd *et al.* 1991). Interestingly, withdrawal of amitriptyline appears to result in elevation of frontal EMG levels in tension-type headache sufferers compared to healthy controls, while no difference was evident during medication (Ellertsen *et al.* 1987).

Regardless of treatment modality, psychology is at work. Treatment effects have been shown to be modestly related to changes in coping strategies and appraisal processes (ter Kuile *et al.* 1995), and response, for example to sumatriptan therapy, is partly determined by pre-treatment quality of life (Litaker *et al.* 1997), while anxiety predicts endurance of symptoms in both migraine and tension-type headache (Guidetti *et al.* 1998).

Both cognitive therapy and behavioural self-management training are effective in decreasing headaches and depressive symptoms (Martin *et al.* 1989). The improvements in symptoms and mood cannot be separated. A meta-analysis has revealed substantial support for the equivalent effectiveness of both propranolol and biofeedback/relaxation training (Holroyd & Penzien 1990). Biofeedback techniques may be no more effective in the short term than relaxation training but both are more effective than control conditions, although this may be a function of therapist contact (Chapman 1986).

Biofeedback may augment long-term improvement after autogenic relaxation training (Cott *et al.* 1992) and, by demonstrating the influence of thoughts and emotions on bodily reactions, may prepare the way for successful cognitive treatment (Kropp *et al.* 1997). A recent study has suggested that a mass-media self-help programme for the behavioural treament of chronic headache may be effective, across diagnostic groups, in reducing frequency and medication use (de Bruijn-Kofman *et al.* 1997).

### How should outcome be assessed?

There is a fundamental difficulty with pain report as both diagnostic criterion and outcome determinant. Pain is subjective. Instruments such as the migraine-specific quality-of-life measure (MSQoL) (Wagner *et al.* 1996) may provide more objective markers of illness, encompassing psychosocial as well as physical functioning.

## The dangers of chronic self-medication

Only 1 per cent of tension-type headache sufferers and 12 per cent of migraine sufferers use prescription medication (Forward *et al.* 1998). A proportion (40 per cent) of patients self-medicating with analgesics experiences no pain relief from the first dose, following the onset of an attack, and therefore takes several doses even though the initial pain might have been rated no higher than in those patients needing only one dose (Passchier *et al.* 1998). This behaviour does not appear to be related to a predisposing addictive personality (Michultka *et al.* 1989). Habituation to the analgesic, intensification of the headache some few hours later, and exacerbation of intensity and frequency for several weeks after discontinuing the medication are features of 'analgesic rebound headache'.

Medication consumption, rather than relieving headache, may actually maintain the pain, and its removal as a pain behaviour reduces headaches in one-third of sufferers (Rapaport 1987). The strategy of analgesic withdrawal is also likely to avoid malpractice risks for the prescribing physician (McAbee 1998), yet withdrawal symptoms, the fear of worsening pain (Saadah 1997) and depression make this a difficult task (Bakal 1997). Withdrawal must be accompanied by the encouragement of increased control over symptoms, for which the clinical psychologist or liaison psychiatrist is ideally placed.

## Recommendations

There is a distinct need for well-designed research into the role of psychological factors in the aetiology and maintenance of headache symptoms. This is particularly the case in tension-type headache, but also in migraine, which, while having a more evident physiological basis, is dependent on illness perceptions and behaviours, for example, medication use.

There is also a case to be made for redirecting attention away from further subclassification and pharmacological development, and towards multidisciplinary treatment programmes for cost-effective and comprehensive management of disabling headaches.

## References

Bahra A & Goadsby P (1998). Co-morbidity of migraine and depression: is there a link? *Progress Neurol Psychiat* **2**, 23–7.

Bakal D (1997). Clinical complexities of managing pain, suffering, and analgesic dependence. *Headache Quarterly* **8**,137–49.

Blomkvist V, Hannerz J, Orth-Gomer K & Theorell T (1997). Coping style and social support in women suffering from cluster headache or migraine. *Psychother Psychosom* **66**, 150–4.

Blumer D & Heilbronn M (1982). Chronic pain as a variant of depressive disease. *J Nerv Ment Dis* **170**, 381–94.

Breslau N (1992). Migraine, suicide ideation and suicide attempts. *Neurology* **42**, 392–5.

Breslau N, Davis G, Schultz L & Patterson E (1994). Migraine and major depression. *Headache* **34**, 387–93.

Breslau N, Chilcoat H & Andreski P (1996). Further evidence of the link between migraine and neuroticism. *Neurology* **47**, 663–7.

Cerbo R, Barbanti P, Fabbrini G, Pascali MP & Cartarci T (1998). Amitriptyline is effective in chronic but not in episodic tension-type headache: pathogenetic implications. *Headache* **38**, 453–7.

Chapman S (1986). A review and clinical perspective on the use of EMG and thermal biofeedback for chronic headaches. *Pain* **27**,1–43.

Coia P & Morley S (1998). Medical reassurance and patients' responses. *J Psychosom Res* **45**, 377–86.

Cott A, Parkinson W, Fabich M, Bedard M & Marlin R (1992). Long-term efficacy of combined relaxation: biofeedback treatments for chronic headache. *Pain* **51**, 49–56.

Davis P, Holm J, Myers T & Suda K (1998). Stress, headache, and physiological disregulation: a time-series analysis of stress in the laboratory. *Headache* **38**, 116–21.

De Benedettis G & Lorenzetti A (1992). Minor stressful life events (daily hassles) in chronic primary headache: relationship with MMPI personality patterns. *Headache* **32**, 330–2.

de Bruijn-Kofman A, van der Wiel H, Groenman N, Sorbi M & Klip E (1997). Effects of a mass media behavioral treatment for chronic headaches. *Headache* **37**, 415–20.

Demjen S, Bakal D & Dunn B (1990). Cognitive correlates of headache intensity and duration. *Headache* **30**, 423–7.

Edmeads J (1998). Why is migraine so common? *Cephalalgia* **18** (Suppl.22), 2–4.

Ellertsen B, Nordby H & Sjaastad O (1987). Psychophysiologic response patterns in tension headache: effects of tricyclic antidepressants. *Cephalalgia* **7**, 55–63.

Faucett J, Gordon N & Levine J (1994). Differences in postoperative pain severity among four ethnic groups. *J Pain Sympt Manage* **9**, 383–9.

Fernandez E & Sheffield J (1996). Relative contributions of life events versus daily hassles to the frequency and intensity of headaches. *Headache* **36**, 595–602.

Forward S, McGrath P, MacKinnon D, Brown T, Swann J & Currie E (1998). Medication patterns of recurrent headache sufferers: a community study. *Cephalalgia* **18**, 146–51.

Gobel H, Hamouz V, Hansen C, Heininger K, Hirsch S, Lindner V, Heuss D & Soyka D (1994). Chronic tension-type headache: amitriptyline reduces clinical headache duration and experimental pain sensitivity but does not alter pericranial muscle activity readings. *Pain* **59**, 241–9.

Goldberg R (1994). Childhood abuse, depression and chronic pain. *Clin J Pain* **109**, 277–81.

Guidetti V, Gaali F, Fabrizi P, Giannantoni AS, Napoli L, Bruni O & Trillo S (1998). Headache and psychiatric comorbidity: clinical aspects and outcome of an 8-year follow-up study. *Cephalalgia* **18**, 455–62.

Hatch J, Schoenfeld L, Boutros N, Seleshi E, Moore P & Cyr-Provost M (1991). Anger and hostility in tension-type headache. *Headache* **31**, 302–4.

Heijmans M (1998). Coping and adaptive outcome in chronic fatigue syndrome: importance of illness cognitions. *J Psychosom Res* **45**, 39–51.

Ho K-H, Ong B & Lee S-C (1997). Headache and self-assessed depression scores in Singapore University undergraduates. *Headache* **37**, 26–30.

Holm J, Bury L & Suda K (1996). The relationship between stress, headache, and the menstrual cycle in young female migraineurs. *Headache* **36**, 531–7.

Holm J, Lamberty K, McSherry W II & Davis P (1997). The stress response in headache sufferers: physiological and psychological reactivity. *Headache* **37**, 221–7.

Holroyd K & Penzien D (1990). Pharmacological versus non-pharmacological prophylaxis of recurrent migraine headache: a meta-analytic review of clinical trials. *Pain* **42**, 1–13.

Holroyd K, Nash J, Pingel J, Cordingley G & Jerome A (1991). A comparison of pharmacological (amitriptyline HCl) and nonpharmacological (cognitive-behavioral) therapies for chronic tension headaches. *J Consult Clin Psychol* **59**, 387–93.

Hursey K & Jacks SD (1992). Fear of pain in recurrent headache sufferers. *Headache* **32**, 283–6.

Jelencsik I (1998). Primary headache and its contemporary management. *Orv Hetil* **139**, 1723–8.

Kohler T & Kosanic S (1992). Are persons with migraine characterized by a high degree of ambition, orderliness and rigidity? *Pain* **48**, 321–3.

Koutantji M, Pearce S & Oakley D (1998). The relationship between gender and family history of pain with current pain experience and awareness of pain in others. *Pain* **77**, 25–31.

Kropp P, Gerber-Wolf D, Keinath-Specht A, Kopal T & Niederberger U (1997). Behavioral treatment in migraine. Cognitive-behavioral therapy and blood-volume-pulse biofeedback: a cross-over study with a two-year followup. *Funct Neurol: New Trends Adapt Behav Disord* **12**, 17–24.

Leijdekkers M & Passchier J (1990). Prediction of migraine using psychophysiological and personality variables. *Headache* **30**, 445–53.

Leijdekkers M, Passchier J, Goudswaard P, Menges L & Orlebeke J (1990). Migraine patients cognitively impaired? *Headache* **30**, 352–8.

Lichstein K, Fischer S, Eakin T, Amberson J, Bertorini T & Hoon P (1991). Psychophysiological parameters of migraine and muscle-contraction headaches. *Headache* **31**, 27–34.

Lipton R, Stewart W, Celentano D & Reed M (1992). Undiagnosed migraine headaches: a comparison of symptom-based and reported physician diagnosis. *Arch Intern Med* **152**, 1273–8.

Litaker D, Solomon G & Genzen B (1997). Using pretreatment quality of life perceptions to predict response to sumatriptan in migraineurs. *Headache* **37**, 630–4.

McAbee G (1998). Malpractice risks associated with prescribing medication for chronic headaches. *Headache* **38**, 53–5.

Marlowe N (1998). Stressful events, appraisal, coping and recurrent headache. *J Clin Psychol* **54**, 247–56.

Martin P, Nathan P, Milech D & van Keppel M (1989). Cognitive therapy vs. self-management training in the treatment of chronic headaches. *Br J Clin Psychol* **28**, 347–61.

Michultka D, Blanchard E, Appelbaum K, Jaccard J & Dentinger M (1989). The refractory headache patient – II: High medication consumption (analgesic rebound) headache. *Behav Res Ther* **27**, 411–20.

Mongini F, Defilippi N & Negro C (1997). Chronic daily headache: a clinical and psychological profile before and after treatment. *Headache* **37**, 83–7.

Passchier J, de Boo M, Quaak J & Brienen J (1996). Health-related quality of life of chronic headache patients is predicted by the emotional component of their pain. *Headache* **36**, 556–60.

Passchier J, Mourik J, Brienen J & Hunfeld J (1998). Cognitions, emotions, and behavior of patients with migraine when taking medication during an attack. *Headache* **38**, 458–64.

Persson B (1997). Growth environment and personality in adult migraineurs and their migraine-free siblings. *Headache* **37**, 159–68.

Peveler R (1998). Understanding medically unexplained symptoms: faster progress in the next century than in this? *J Psychosom Res* **45**, 93–7.

Pfaffenrath V, Diener HC, Isler H, Meyer C, Scholz E, Taneri Z, Wessely P, Zaiser-Kaschel H, Haase W & Fischer W (1993). Effectiveness and tolerance of amitriptyline oxide in chronic tension-type headache – a multicenter double-blind study versus amitriptyline versus placebo. *Nervenarzt* **64**, 114–20.

Rapaport A (1987). *Characteristics and treatment of analgesic rebound headache*. Springer, New York.

Rasmussen BK & Olesen J (1994). Epidemiology of migraine and tension-type headache. *Curr Opinion Neurol* **7**, 264–71.

Rasmussen BK, Jensen R & Olesen J (1992). Impact of headache on sickness absence and utilisation of medical services: a Danish population study. *J Epidemiol Comm Health* **46**, 443–6.

Saadah H (1997). Headache fear. *J Okla State Med Ass* **90**, 179–84.

Solomon G (1997). Evolution of the measurement of quality of life in migraine. *Neurology* **48** (Suppl.3), 10–15.

Spierings E, Sorbi M, Maassen G & Honkoop P (1997). Psychophysical precedents of migraine in relation to the time of onset of the headache: the migraine time line. *Headache* **37**, 217–20.

Stronks D, Tulen J, Verheij R, Boomsma F, Fekkes D, Pepplinkhuizen L, Mantel G & Passchier J (1998). Serotonergic, catecholaminergic, and cardiovascular reactions to mental stress in female migraine patients. A controlled study. *Headache* **38**, 270–80.

ter Kuile M, Spinhoven P, Linssen AC & van Houwelingen H (1995). Cognitive coping and appraisal processes in the treatment of chronic headaches. *Pain* **64**, 257–64.

Ulrich V, Russell MB, Jensen R & Olesen J (1996). A comparison of tension-type headache in migraineurs and in non-migraineurs: a population study. *Pain* **67**, 501–6.

Verri A, Proietti Cecchini A, Galli C, Granella F, Sandrini G & Nappi G (1998). Psychiatric comorbidity in chronic daily headache. *Cephalalgia* **18** (Suppl.21), 45–9.

von Korff M & Simon G (1996). The relationship between pain and depression. *Br J Psychiat* **168**, S101–8.

Voudouris N, Peck C & Coleman G (1990). The role of conditioning and verbal expectancy in the placebo response. *Pain* **43**, 121–8.

Wagner T, Patrick D, Galer B & Berzon R (1996). A new instrument to assess the long-term quality of life effects from migraine: development and psychometric testing of the MSQoL. *Headache* **36**, 484–92.

Wall PD (1994). The placebo and the placebo response. In *Textbook of pain* 3rd edn (ed. PD Wall & R Melzack). Churchill Livingstone, London.

Ziegler D & Paolo A (1996). Self-reported disability due to headache: a comparison of clinic patients and controls. *Headache* **36**, 476–80.

PART 2

# Evidence and Treatment

Chapter 6

# Treatment of headache and prophylaxis

*Andrew J Dowson*

## Introduction

Migraine is a common condition – it is thought to affect around 15–18 per cent of women and 6 per cent of men (Rasmussen *et al.* 1991; Lipton & Stewart 1994), although estimates vary (Breslau *et al.* 1991; Henry *et al.* 1992; Gobel *et al.* 1994; O'Brien *et al.* 1994). A firm understanding of the presentations of migraine will improve diagnosis; accurate diagnosis is the foundation for effective prescribing. The introduction of the 5-HT$_1$ agonists has increased treatment options in migraine and provides an opportunity to re-appraise management strategies. This chapter will consider the relative role of acute and prophylactic regimes and outline logical selection criteria for 5-HT$_1$ agonists in clinical practice.

Sinister symptoms are outside the scope of this chapter but, in reality, general practitioners (GPs) do worry about misdiagnosing presenting symptoms of serious underlying pathology. They should, however, be reassured that these presentations are extremely rare. It is also important to remember that those patients whose management is unsuccessful may have been misdiagnosed and therefore given inappropriate treatment.

Many of our preconceived ideas about migraine are in fact mistaken. Some GPs believe that a typical migraineur is a woman in her 50s who experiences as many as four attacks per month, whereas, in reality, the average frequency of attacks is one or two per month and most sufferers are between the ages of 25 and 55 (Cull *et al.* 1992; Glaxo Wellcome 1992; Lipton & Stewart 1994). Only a minority of sufferers (about one in five) experience more than 40 attacks per year (Bates *et al.* 1997). GPs should be aware that frequent attacks may indicate other diagnoses and, in particular, they should know about the possibility of the chronic daily headache syndrome (CDH). Patients with this condition require specific management that is different from the one appropriate for migraine, and they may benefit from the intervention of a headache specialist in order to break up the headache pattern.

## Diagnosis of headache

Migraine is most commonly diagnosed using the International Headache Society classification (Box 6.1). A more modern approach, however, might include questions relating to the disruption of normal activity and quality of life. These are much less affected by episodic tension-type headache, the symptoms of which are the inverse of migraine (Box 6.2).

> **Box 6.1** Diagnostic pointers for migraine
>
> Attacks last from 4 to 72 hours
>
> Headache is at least two of the following:
>
> – unilateral
> – pulsating
> – of moderate/severe intensity
> – aggravated by routine activities
>
> Accompanying symptoms may include photophobia, phonophobia and nausea, with or without vomiting
>
> Patients are usually symptom-free between attacks

*Source:* Adapted from Headache Classification Committee of the International Headache Society (1988)

> **Box 6.2** Diagnostic pointers for muscle contraction/episodic tension headache
>
> May persist for longer periods than migraine
>
> Headache is at least two of the following:
>
> – bilateral
> – non-pulsating
> – of mild/moderate intensity
> – not aggravated by routine activities
>
> Any features of sensory sensitivity (nausea, photophobia, phonophobia) more likely to suggest migraine, not tension headache

*Source:* Adapted from Headache Classification Committee of the International Headache Society (1988)

Chronic daily headache is defined as headache being present on the majority of days in the month, typically over a period of six months or longer. It is characterised by a combination of background muscle contraction-type symptoms with superimposed migraine (Figure 6.1).

The patient may have had migraine in the past and experienced a difficult patch of high-frequency attacks, prompting them to increase their intake of analgesics. This in turn tends to fuel chronic daily headache. Codeine is the most commonly implicated drug in the UK, although simple analgesics and ergotamine have also been reported. The new headache pattern then becomes far more disabling than straightforward migraine. Risk factors appear to include not only a past medical history of migraine and analgesic intake but previous head or neck injuries.

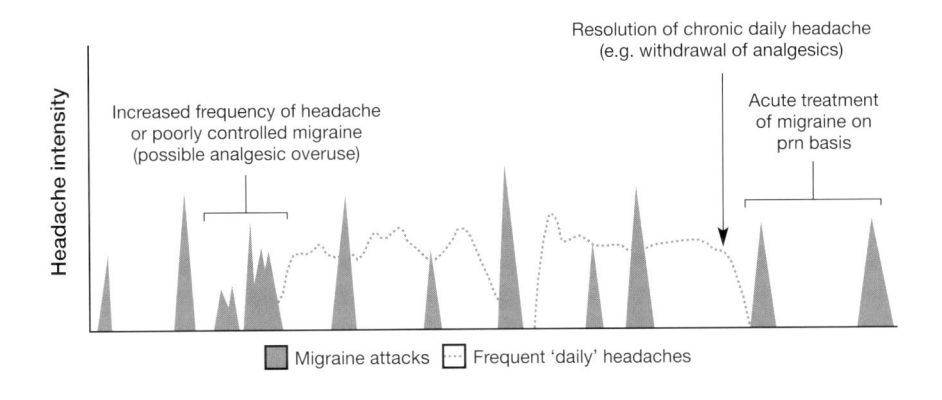

**Figure 6.1** Chronic daily headache syndrome. (Adapted from MIPCA Guidelines, Synergy Medical Education 1997)

## Management of headache

The aim of management for chronic daily headache should be for the patient to downgrade to their previous acute headache and this often requires a combination of physical methods to neck and shoulders, such as exercises or formal physiotherapy, the avoidance of analgesics and ergotamine and the use of regular medication, usually drawn from the antidepressant and anti-epileptic groups. When considering prophylaxis in migraine, it is critical that chronic daily headache is not inadvertently missed.

### The changing nature of migraine management

Before the advent of 5-HT$_1$ agonists, analgesics and ergot were the principal migraine treatments but, although they were effective in some patients, they left considerable room for improvement. Their limited efficacy with the potential for chronic side-effects may have been behind the low threshold for initiating prophylactic treatment at two or more migraine attacks per month (Bates *et al.* 1997).

The goalposts for migraine treatments have now changed. The identification of the 5-HT$_1$ receptor, its involvement in migraine and the subsequent development of the 5-HT$_1$ agonists have increased the options for effective acute treatment of migraine. As a result, it is now appropriate to increase the threshold for initiating prophylaxis to four or more attacks per month.

A threshold of number of attacks for the initiation of prophylaxis is only a guideline and not a gold standard. Individual patients should be considered on their own merits: ultimately, it is the patient and not their medical adviser who manages their condition. The patient must, therefore, be involved in decision making on therapeutic intervention. It may be that a patient who has a low attack rate may have a long duration of attack which never completely clears with acute therapies. Such a patient may prefer to take

**Table 6.1** Response to propranolol in trials

| Authors | Number of patients | Dose | Response rate (% of patients) Propranolol | Response rate (% of patients) Placebo |
|---|---|---|---|---|
| Diener et al 1996* | 214 | 40 mg tds | 42 | 31 (NS) |
| Gerber et al 1991** | 58 | 160 mg/day | 32 | – |
| Gerber et al 1995† | 62 | 120 mg/day then 160 mg/day | 53 | 18 (significant difference) |
| Johnson et al. (1986)* | 17 | 40 mg tds | 35 | 12 (P<0.01) |
| Kangasniemi et al. (1994)‡ | 33 | 80 mg bd | 48 | – |
| Ludin (1989)* | 59 | 40 mg tds | 50 | – |
| Olesen (1984)‡ | 53 | 40 mg bd | 30 | – |
| Sudilovsky et al. (1987)* | 98 | 80 mg bd | 19 | – |
| Tfelt-Hansen et al. (1984)* | 81 | 80 mg bd | 60 | 30 (P=0.01) |

*Response defined as:*
\* >50 per cent reduction in migraine attack frequency
\*\* Significant reduction in migraine attack frequency
† 50 per cent reduction in days with migraine
‡ 50 per cent reduction in severity (intensity x frequency)
NS = not significant; bd = twice a day; tds = three times a day

medication on a regular basis to reduce the frequency of attacks. Another may find no acute treatment to be effective so that it may be necessary to introduce prophylaxis at an earlier stage.

The original guidelines for the introduction of prophylaxis (two or more attacks of migraine per month) were in fact not based upon any specific scientific data but, with the introduction of the triptans, more acute and less prophylactic therapies are now being used in the management of migraine.

## Assessment of prophylactic agents

Factors influencing the choice of prophylactic medication include efficacy, tolerability, convenience and cost. When pizotifen and propranolol, the drugs which are mainly used as prophylaxis in the UK, are measured against these criteria, they may not be particularly effective.

Efficacy is usually defined as a reduction of at least 50 per cent in the frequency of attacks (Bates et al. 1997); using this criterion, both propranolol and pizotifen are only efficacious in about half the number of patients taking these agents for prophylaxis (see Tables 6.1 and 6.2). Neither drug appears to reduce the severity of breakthrough attacks and, therefore, the patient will also need to have an effective acute treatment available (Bates et al. 1997).

**Table 6.2** Response to pizotifen in trials

| Authors | Number of patients | Dose | Response rate (% of patients)* Pizotifen | Response rate (% of patients)* Placebo |
| --- | --- | --- | --- | --- |
| Arthur et al. (1971) | 104 | 3 mg/day | 40 | 12 |
| Capildeo & Rose (1982) | 17 | 0.5 mg tds or 1.5 mg nocte | 47 | (active comparator) |
| Graham (1968) | 52 |  | 52 | Not reported |
| Hughes & Foster (1971) | 26 | 1 mg tds | 35 | Reported as NS |
| Lance & Anthony (1968) | 50 | 3 mg/day | 48 | 36 (NS) |
| Lance et al. (1970) | 290 | 1.5–4 mg/day | 50 | 32 |
| Sjaastad & Stensrud (1969) | 20 | 1 mg qds | 45 | Not reported |

* Response defined as a 50 per cent reduction in migraine attack frequency
NS = not significant; tds = three times a day; qds = four times a day

Both propranolol and pizotifen are associated with chronic side-effects (Bates et al. 1997). Patients taking pizotifen may experience drowsiness or lethargy and an estimated 40 per cent of patients will gain weight – usually 2–4 kg (Speight & Avery 1972). With propranolol and other beta-blockers, common side-effects include arterial hypotension, muscle fatigue, violent dreams, bronchospasm and impotence (Diener & Limmroth 1994). Up to 40 per cent of subjects have reported fatigue in some studies (Nadelmann et al. 1986; Gerber et al. 1991).

Many patients may not understand the rationale for prophylaxis – if they only have one attack per month, why should they take a tablet every day? Some patients may, therefore, be less likely to comply with a prophylactic regimen than with acute therapy taken at the time of an attack. Convenience is reduced still further by the need to take extra acute therapy for breakthrough attacks (Bates et al. 1997).

As soon as a prophylactic agent is introduced, it is important for the patient to realise that the medication is not in fact designed to cure their migraine but to reduce rather than prevent all their attacks. The patient must be involved in decision making with regard to the therapeutic options, since the balance between efficacy and side-effects of individual medications will obviously affect patient preference. An acute drug can be cost-effective and patients may well have the bonus of fewer long-term side-effects. Prophylaxis with pizotifen (1.5 mg/day) costs approximately £8 for 28 days of treatment (MIMS 1998). If the patient suffers two attacks per month, one of these attacks may be prevented at the cost of £8; however, both attacks could be treated with a 5-HT$_1$ agonist for the same amount (Figure 6.2). It should be remembered that, in pricing prophylaxis, the cost of prescribing acute therapy for breakthrough attacks must also be taken into account.

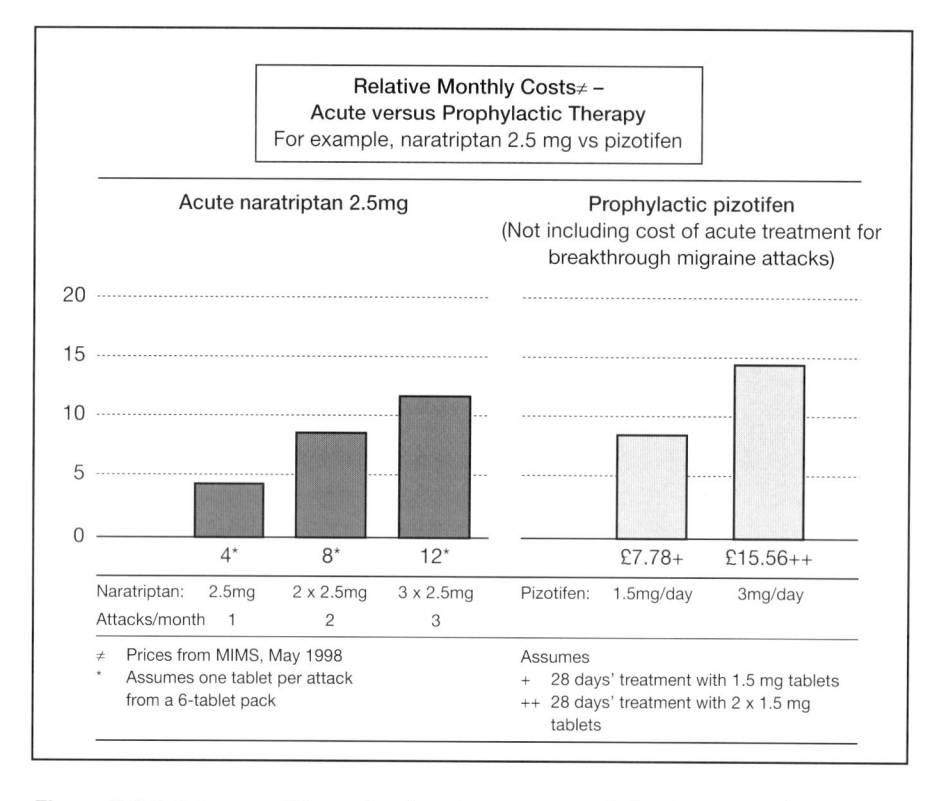

**Figure 6.2** Relative monthly costs of acute versus prophylactic therapy (Prices from MIMS (1998))

## Management of patients

Prophylactic therapy may be considered appropriate if a patient is experiencing four or more attacks per month. It should be remembered, however, that acute therapy including 5-HT$_1$ agonists is now available and effective without prophylaxis for the majority of patients. Over 50 per cent of patients respond to simple analgesics, with or without gastric motility anti-emetics.

The frequency and severity of migraine vary and a patient may experience 'bad patches' even when on prophylaxis. These cases should be reviewed on a 3–6 monthly basis.

Prophylaxis withdrawal should be considered after several months:

- if the medication appears ineffective;
- if it is causing side-effects;
- if the attacks have come under control.

A strategy for the management of migraine is outlined in Figures 6.3 and 6.4.

The importance of including the patient in management decisions cannot be over-stressed. A package of care needs to be developed which is specifically tailored to the individual patient's needs, and this should include:

- the avoidance of trigger factors when they can be identified;
- acute intervention for breakthrough attacks;
- the use of prophylactic agents in high attack frequency patients.

In practical terms, the decision about prophylaxis is usually taken with the primary care physician (GP) when it has been ascertained that simple analgesics, plus or minus a gastric motility drug, taken early in an attack, have proved ineffective.

## Which triptan – the available evidence

This chapter has so far centred upon the relative role of acute treatment and prophylactic medication. The remainder will be focused on factors influencing the choice of $5\text{-HT}_1$ agonists in general practice. At the time of writing, there are four available drugs within this class: sumatriptan, zolmitriptan, naratriptan and rizatriptan.

The $5\text{-HT}_1$ agonists are convenient for patients because they are available not only as tablets but also in subcutaneous, intranasal and fast-melt formulations and need only be taken when an attack occurs. In contrast to the treatments used for migraine prophylaxis, the $5\text{-HT}_1$ agonists are highly effective in the acute treatment of migraine, the majority of patients responding at about four hours (Lowy & Cady 1996; Gijsman *et al.* 1997; Göbel *et al.* 1997; Mathew *et al.* 1997; Pfaffenrath *et al.* 1998).

The $5\text{-HT}_1$ agonists are thought to act partly by stimulating receptors on the cranial blood vessels. This produces cranial vasoconstriction, which counteracts the vasodilation which is believed to give rise to migraine headache. They may also inhibit trigeminal nerve activity, thereby inhibiting the release of vaso-active peptides that cause neurogenic inflammation. There are two potential sites of action on the trigeminal nerve, in the periphery and also at the trigeminal nucleus, which is on the brain side of the blood-brain barrier. It is thought that sumatriptan cannot cross the blood-brain barrier because of its poor lipophilicity and, therefore, this may inhibit its ability to influence the trigeminal nerve. Zolmitriptan, rizatriptan and naratriptan are more lipophilic and, therefore, better able to cross the blood-brain barrier. It has been suggested that this dual mode of action may offer advantage in terms of efficacy, although published comparative trials versus sumatriptan have yielded little evidence to support this (Cutler *et al.* 1995; Sargent *et al.* 1995; Fazekas 1997; Göbel *et al.* 1997; MDS 1998).

It may be that, in certain circumstances, a particular drug may be more effective than another and it is necessary to consider the varying profiles from clinical trial data so that logical selection criteria can be established. Available data comparing the triptans are, however, limited. Any comparative study tends to include sumatriptan, there being no direct studies between the newer agents. It can, therefore, be difficult for the

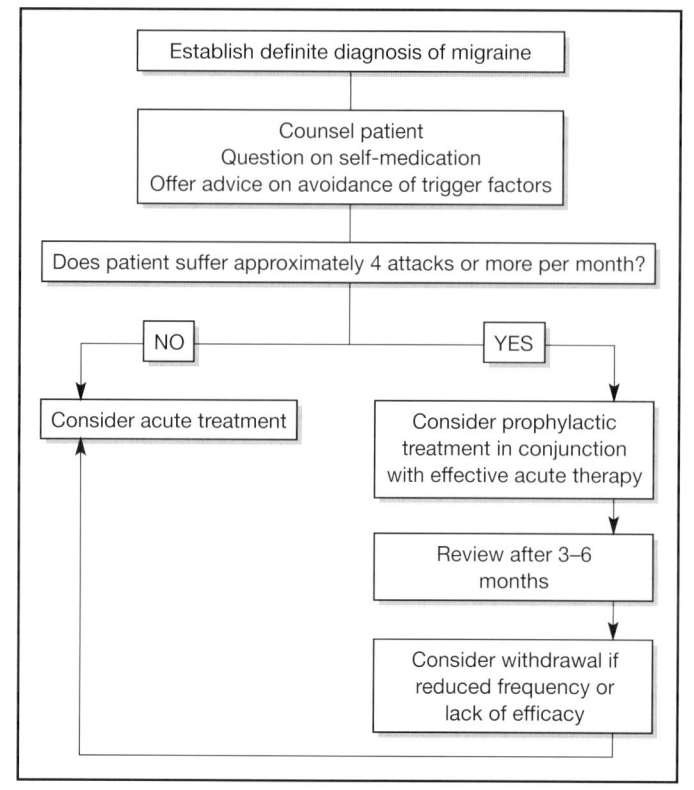

```
┌─────────────────────────────────────────────────┐
│         Establish definite diagnosis of migraine │
│                         │                        │
│                Counsel patient                   │
│           Question on self-medication            │
│      Offer advice on avoidance of trigger factors│
│                         │                        │
│   Does patient suffer approximately 4 attacks or more per month? │
│              NO                YES               │
│               │                 │                │
│     Consider acute treatment    Consider prophylactic │
│                                 treatment in conjunction │
│                                 with effective acute therapy │
│                                 │                │
│                        Review after 3–6 months   │
│                                 │                │
│                        Consider withdrawal if    │
│                        reduced frequency or     │
│                        lack of efficacy         │
└─────────────────────────────────────────────────┘
```

Patients with less frequent but more prolonged attacks may warrant prophylaxis if their migraines are unresponsive to 5-HT$_1$ agonists

**Figure 6.3** A strategy for when to use prophylactic or acute therapy for migraine (*Source*: Bates *et al.* (1997))

GP to make a decision as to which 5-HT$_1$ agonist to prescribe first. In addition to efficacy, other factors need to be considered, such as side-effects, which are associated with all medications (patient tolerability differs between various agents), and cost.

Comparison of different studies has recently been undertaken using therapeutic gain or 'number needed to treat' analyses. Methodology regarding both these measures are discussed elsewhere in the publication (see Chapter 7). However, there are some difficulties with the analyses as studies undertaken at different times and with different populations using different methodology may represent populations which should not be directly compared.

Patients would prefer their treatment to be effective as soon as possible, and all available 5-HT$_1$ agonists have been shown to be effective for some patients within an hour of administration (some trial evidence exists for 30-minute response to sumatriptan and rizatriptan) (Diener & Klein 1996; Martin 1996).

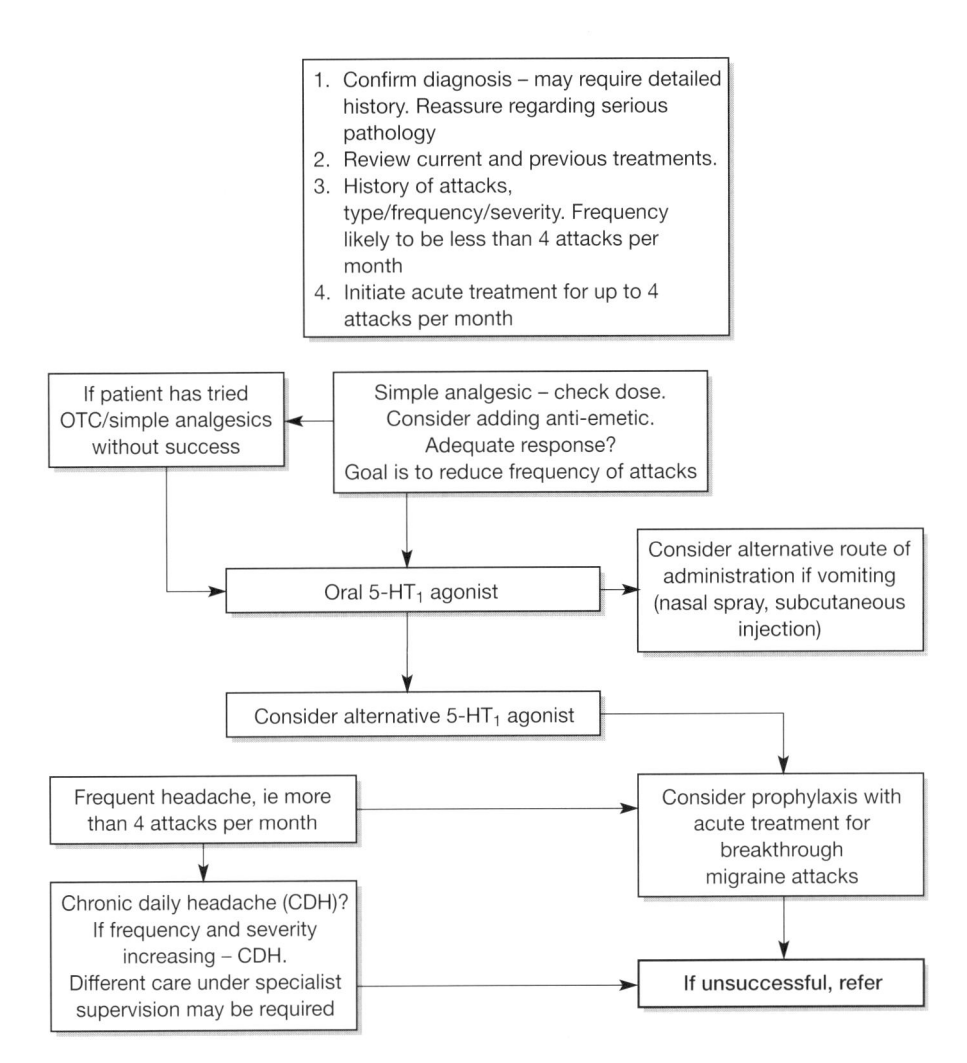

## Figure 6.4 Migraine management strategy

1. Confirm diagnosis – may require detailed history. Reassure regarding serious pathology
2. Review current and previous treatments.
3. History of attacks, type/frequency/severity. Frequency likely to be less than 4 attacks per month
4. Initiate acute treatment for up to 4 attacks per month

- If patient has tried OTC/simple analgesics without success
- Simple analgesic – check dose. Consider adding anti-emetic. Adequate response? Goal is to reduce frequency of attacks
- Oral 5-HT$_1$ agonist
- Consider alternative route of administration if vomiting (nasal spray, subcutaneous injection)
- Consider alternative 5-HT$_1$ agonist
- Frequent headache, ie more than 4 attacks per month
- Chronic daily headache (CDH)? If frequency and severity increasing – CDH. Different care under specialist supervision may be required
- Consider prophylaxis with acute treatment for breakthrough migraine attacks
- If unsuccessful, refer

Table 6.3 represents the comparison of headache response (defined as moderate or severe pain reducing to mild or absent pain) at two hours for the 5-HT$_1$ agonists. All available published data have been analysed and a range of results shown for both the index drug and the placebo group.

It should be remembered that patients involved in clinical trials must wait until the headache is moderate before dosing and they represent a group of patients who are perhaps regarded as difficult as they have a higher frequency of attacks than the general population. These studies usually comprise groups seen in secondary care. The recorded response rates do not, therefore, reflect normal primary care clinical practice.

**Table 6.3** Comparison of headache response at two hours for 5-HT$_1$ agonists: two-hour response rates

|  | % | Placebo (%) |
| --- | --- | --- |
| Sumatriptan 50 mg | 49–54 | 17–26 |
| Sumatriptan 100 mg | 46–67 | 10–31 |
| Naratriptan 2.5 mg | 40–52 | 22–31 |
| Zolmitriptan 2.5 mg | 62–65 | 34–36 |
| Zolmitriptan 5 mg | 62–67 | 15–34 |
| Rizatriptan 10 mg | 48–77 | 18–40 |

The overall impression is of great overlap between the various agents with placebo averaging between 25 and 30 per cent. Analysis at 4 hours would show similar overlap but the rates for both active drug and placebo would be higher (Nappi *et al.* 1984; Goadsby *et al.* 1991; The Oral Sumatriptan Dose-Defining Study Group (1991); Dahlof *et al.* 1995; Rapoport *et al.* 1995; Tfelt-Hansen *et al.* 1995; Visser *et al.* 1996a; Dahlof *et al.* 1997; Glaxo Wellcome 1997b; Glaxo Wellcome 1997c; Kramer *et al.* 1997; Solomon *et al.* 1997; Zeneca 1997; Teall *et al.* 1998).

Another area for comparison is the duration of action, termed 'headache recurrence', in this field. This is when a patient has response but within 24 hours there is recurrence of headache. Different studies do use differing definitions of recurrent headache, which again makes direct comparison difficult.

Table 6.4 shows the range of results available for the various drugs and, again, overlap is demonstrated (Goadsby *et al.* 1991; The Oral Sumatriptan Dose-Defining Study Group 1991; Martin 1996; Glaxo Wellcome 1997a; Göbel *et al.* 1997; Kramer *et al.* 1997).

Naratriptan has a longer half-life than sumatriptan, zolmitriptan or rizatriptan (Diener & Klein 1996; Visser *et al.* 1996b; Visser *et al.* 1997; Teall *et al.* 1998) but this pharmacokinetic property alone is not thought to determine time to recurrence. Naratriptan does, however, have a reduced rate of recurrence compared to sumatriptan (Göbel *et al.* 1997).

Side-effects regarded as characteristic of 5-HT$_1$ agonists include: chest discomfort, dizziness and nausea.

Naratriptan is the only available 5-HT$_1$ agonist with a side-effect profile similar to placebo in clinical trials (Fazekas 1997).

Interactions between various triptans have not been described because the drugs have not been studied when used concomitantly in an attack. This should, therefore, not be recommended. Similarly, ergotamine has never been used concomitantly with a triptan and should also be avoided. With regard to preventive agents, monoamineoxydase inhibitors (MAOIs) have potential interaction with all but naratriptan. However, as MAOIs are rarely used for migraine prophylaxis in this

**Table 6.4** Duration of action (headache recurrence)

|  | % |
|---|---|
| Naratriptan 2.5 mg | 17–28 |
| Sumatriptan 100 mg | 30–40 |
| Zolmitriptan 5 mg | 22–36 |
| Rizatriptan 10 mg | 33–47 |

country, they do not constitute a clinical problem. The selective serotonin re-uptake inhibitors (SSRIs) are contra-indicated with sumatriptan, and this is perhaps a legacy of the data available at launch for sumatriptan as it was felt potential side-effects may worsen by elongating the length of action of sumatriptan with an SSRI. However, this has later appeared not to be the case, and many clinicians advocate the use of the drugs concomitantly off licence. Rizatriptan shares the same metabolic pathway as propranolol and, for this reason, a 5 mg dose (standard dose 10 mg) must be used if propranolol is also prescribed.

The only other major interaction is lithium with sumatriptan and this is, therefore, contra-indicated. Clearly, this is not a problem with migraine but, in cluster headache, it could represent a difficulty.

Direct comparison studies are needed between the various triptans to ascertain the relative advantages or disadvantages in given situations. Standardisation of endpoints would also be useful, while it is important that we develop analyses which reflect both clinical practice and clinically relevant endpoints in terms of patient agenda.

## Conclusion

There is now a wealth of treatments available for patients with migraine and GPs should be striving to achieve an individual management plan which minimises the impact of a patient's attacks while causing the fewest possible side-effects. The aim is for patients to feel in control of their migraine rather than that their condition is controlling them.

### *References*
Arthur GP & Hornabrook RW (1971). The treatment of migraine with BC-105 (pizotifen): a double-blind trial. *NZ Med J* **464**, 5–9.
Bates D, Bradbury P, Capildeo R *et al.* (1997). *Migraine management guidelines: a strategy for the modern management of migraine*. Synergy Medical Education, London.
Breslau N, Davis GC & Andreski P (1991). Migraine, psychiatric disorders and suicide attempts: an epidemiological study of young adults. *Psychiatry Res* **37**, 11–23.
Capildeo R & Rose FC (1982). Single-dose pizotifen, 1.5 mg nocte; a new approach in the prophylaxis of migraine. *Headache* **22**, 272–5.

Cull RE, Wells NEJ & Miocevich ML (1992). The economic cost of migraine. *Brit J Med Econ* **2**, 103–15.

Cutler N, Mushet GR, Davis R *et al.* (1995). Oral sumatriptan for the acute treatment of migraine; evaluation of three dosage strengths. *Neurology* **45**(Suppl.7), S5–S9.

Dahlof C, Diener HC, Goadby PJ *et al.* (1995). A multicentre, double-blind, placebo-controlled, dose-range finding study to investigate the efficacy and safety of oral doses of 311C90 in the acute treatment of migraine. *Headache* **35**, 292, Abstr.19.

Dahlof C, Winter P, Whitehouse H & Hassani H (1997). Randomized, double-blind, placebo-controlled comparison of oral naratriptan and oral sumatriptan in the acute treatment of migraine. *Neurology* **48**, A85–A86.

Diener HC & Klein KB (1996). The first comparison of the efficacy and safety of 311C90 and sumatriptan in the treatment of migraine. Poster presented at the 3rd Congress of the European Headache Federation, Sardinia.

Diener HC & Limmroth V (1994). The management of migraine. *Rev Contemp Pharmacother* **5**, 271–84.

Diener HC, Föl M, Iaccario C *et al.* (1996). Cyclandelate in the prophylaxis of migraine: a randomised parallel, double-blind study in comparison with placebo and propranolol. *Cephalalgia* **16**, 441–7.

Fazekas A (1997). The efficacy, tolerability and safety of oral sumatriptan 50 mg in the acute treatment of migraine. Presented at the 8th International Headache Congress, Amsterdam.

Gerber WD, Diener HC, Scholz E & Niederberger U (1991). Responders and non-responders to metoprolol, propranolol and nifedipine treatment in migraine prophylaxis; a dose-ranging study based on time series analysis. *Cephalalgia* **11**, 37–45.

Gerber WD, Schellenberg R, Thom M *et al.* (1995). Cyclandelate versus propranolol in the prophylaxis of migraine – a double-blind placebo-controlled study. *Funct Neurol* **10**, 27–35.

Gijsman H, Kramer MS, Sargent J *et al.* (1997). Double-blind, placebo-controlled, dose-finding study of rizatriptan (MK-462) in the acute treatment of migraine. *Cephalalgia* **17**, 647–51.

Glaxo Wellcome UK Limited (1992). *Migraine: the patient's perspective*. Data on file.

Glaxo Wellcome (1997a). *Imigran tablets: summary of product characteristics*.

Glaxo Wellcome (1997b). *Naramig tablets: summary of product characteristics*.

Glaxo Wellcome (1997c). Data on file (S2WB3002).

Goadsby PJ, Zagami AS, Donnan GA *et al.* (1991). Oral sumatriptan in acute migraine. *Lancet* **338**, 782–3.

Gobel H, Petersen-Braun M & Soyka D (1994). The epidemiology of headache in Germany: a nationwide survey of a representative sample on the basis of the headache classification of the International Headache Society. *Cephalalgia* **14**, 97–106.

Göbel H, Boswell B, Winter PDO'B *et al.* (1997). A comparison of the efficacy and tolerability of naratriptan and sumatriptan among migraineurs with history of frequent (<50% of attacks) headache recurrence. Poster presented at the 8th International Headache Congress, Amsterdam.

Graham JR (1968). *Headache rounds*. The Faulkner Hospital, June 26.

Headache Classification Committee of the International Headache Society (1988). Classification and diagnostic criteria for headache disorders, cranial neuralgias and facial pain. *Cephalgia* **8**(Suppl.7), 1–96.

Henry P, Michel P. Brochet B *et al.* (1992). A nationwide survey of migraine in France: prevalence and clinical features in adults. *Cephalalgia* **12**, 229–37.

Hughes RC & Foster JB (1971). BC-105 in the prophylaxis of migraine. *Curr Ther Res* **13**(1), 63–8.

Johnson RH, Hornabrook RW & Lambie DG (1986). Comparison of mefanamic acid and propranolol with placebo in migraine prophylaxis. *Acta Neurol Scand* **73**, 490–2.

Johnson RH, Hornabrook Gijsman H, Kramer MS, Sargent J *et al.* (1997). Double-blind, placebo-controlled, dose-finding study of rizatriptan (MK-462) in the acute treatment of migraine. *Cephalalgia* **17**, 647–51.

Kangasniemi P & Hedman C (1984). Metoprolol and propranolol in the prophylactic treatment of classical and common migraine: a double-blind study. *Cephalalgia* **4**, 91–6.

Kramer MS, Matzura-Wolfe D, Getson A *et al.* (1997). Placebo-controlled, double-blind study of rizatriptan in multiple attacks of migraine. Poster 24, presented at the 39th AASH, New York.

Lance JW & Anthony M (1968). Clinical trial of a new serotonin antagonist, BC-105, in the prevention of migraine. *Med J Aust* **1**, 54.

Lance JW, Anthony M & Somerville B (1970). Comparative trial of serotonin antagonists in the management of migraine. *Br Med J* **2**, 327.

Lipton RB & Stewart WF (1994). The epidemiology of migraine. *Eur Neurol* **34**(Suppl.2), 6–11.

Lowy M & Cady R (1996). 2.5 mg of 311C90 in the acute treatment of migraine: efficacy and safety. Poster presented at the 2nd Congress of the European Federation of Neurological Societies.

Ludin HP (1989). Flunarizine and propranolol in the treatment of migraine. *Headache* **29**, 218–23.

Martin GR (1996). Inhibition of the trigeminovascular system with 5-HT$_{1D}$ drugs: selectivity targeting additional sites of action. *Eur Neurol* **36**(Suppl.2), 13–18.

Mathew NT, Asgharnejad M, Paykamian MD *et al.* on behalf of the naratriptan S2WA3003 study group (1997). Naratriptan is effective and well tolerated in the acute treatment of migraine. *Neurology* **49**, 1485–90.

MIMS (1998), July.

MSD (1998). *Maxalt: summary of product characteristics,* June.

Nadelmann JW, Stevens J & Saper JR (1986). Propranolol in the prophylaxis of migraine. *Headache* **26**, 175–82.

Nappi G, Sicuteri F, Byrne M *et al.* (1984). Oral sumatriptan compared with placebo in the acute treatment of migraine. *J Neurol* **241**, 138–44.

O'Brien B, Goeree R & Streiner D (1994). Prevalence of migraine headache in Canada: a population-based survey. *Int J Epidemiol* **23**, 1020–6.

Olesen JE (1984). Metoprolol and propranolol in migraine prophylaxis: a double-blind multicentre study. *Acta Neurol Scand* **70**, 160–8.

The Oral Sumatriptan Dose-Defining Study Group (1991). Sumatriptan – an oral dose-defining study. *Eur Neurol* **31**, 300–5.

Pfaffenrath V, Cunin G, Sjonell G & Prendergast S (1998). Efficacy and safety of sumatriptan tablets (25mg, 50mg and 100mg) in the acute treatment of migraine; defining the optimum doses of oral sumatriptan. *Headache* **38**, 184–90.

Rapoport AM, Cady RK, Matther AN *et al.* (1995). Optimizing the oral dose of 311C90 in the acute treatment of migraine. *Cephalalgia* **15**(Suppl.14), 221, Abstr. P19.

Rasmussen BK, Jensen R, Schroll M & Olesen J (1991). Epidemiology of headache in a general population – a prevalence study. *J Clin Epidemiol* **44**, 1147–57.

Sargent J, Kirchner JR, David R & Kirkhart B (1995). Oral sumatriptan is effective and well tolerated for the acute treatment of migraine; results of a multicentre study. *Neurology* **45** (Suppl.7), S10–S14.

Sjaastad O & Stensrud P (1969). Appraisal of BC-105 in migraine prophylaxis. *Acta Neurol Scand* **45**, 594.

Solomon GD, Cady RK, Klapper KA & Saper JR (1997). 2.5 mg 311C90 (Zomig, zolmitriptan) is clinically effective in treating migraine: clinical efficacy and improvement in activity. Presented at the AAN Boston.

Speight TM & Avery GS (1972). Pizotifen (BC-105): a review of its pharmacological properties and its therapeutic efficacy in vascular headaches. *Drugs* **3**, 159–203.

Sudilovsky A, Elkind AH, Ryan RE Sr *et al.* (1987). Comparative efficacy of nadolol and propranolol in the management of migraine. *Headache* **27**, 421–6.

Teall J, Tuchman M, Cutler N *et al.* (1998). Rizatriptan (MAXALT) for the acute treatment of migraine recurrence. A placebo-controlled, outpatient study. *Headache* **38**, 281–7.

Tfelt-Hansen P, Standnes B, Kangasniemi P *et al.* (1984). Timolol vs propranolol vs placebo in common migraine prophylaxis: a double-blind multicentre study. *Acta Neurol Scand* **69**, 1–8.

Tfelt-Hansen P, Henry P, Mulder LJ *et al.* (1995). The effectiveness of combined oral lysine acetylsalicylate and metoclopramide compared with oral sumatriptan for migraine. *Lancet* **346**, 923–6.

Visser WH, Klein KB, Cox RC *et al.* (1996a). 311C90, a new central and peripherally acting 5-HT$_{1D}$ receptor agonist in the acute oral treatment of migraine: a double-blind, placebo-controlled, dose-range finding study. *Neurology* **46**, 522–6.

Visser WH, Terwindt GM, Reines SA *et al.* (1996b). Rizatriptan versus sumatriptan in the acute treatment of migraine. *Arch Neurol* **53**, 1132–7.

Visser WH, Teall JH, Malbecq W *et al.* (1997). Early onset of action of rizatriptan versus sumatriptan in the acute treatment of migraine. *Headache* **37**, 319–320.

Zeneca (1997). *Zomig: summary of product characteristics*, April.

Chapter 7

# Clinical effectiveness of migraine therapy: the number needed to treat and therapeutic gain methods

*Peter J Goadsby*

## Introduction

The evaluation of new medicines for headache is an important issue from several perspectives. The evaluation of new medicines with regard to pharmaco-economic benefit is explicitly covered in Chapter 8; in this chapter I will address some of the various methods currently used to assess compounds against placebo and then between each other. The issues will be illustrated by the triptan class of drugs (Goadsby 1998a), which are used in the acute treatment of migraine (Lance & Goadsby 1998). The review is divided into a discussion of endpoint measures and then a consideration of some summary measures – the therapeutic gain and number needed to treat (NNT).

### Endpoints in migraine clinical trials

The issue of which endpoints to use is somewhat vexed. Some options are listed in Table 7.1. The list is not exhaustive but illustrates the problem. In essence, there is a competition between the need for scientific rigour, particularly in establishing efficacy in a new class of medicines – the core problem that faced the sumatriptan development team – and the need to provide clinically useful information, which is a more pressing need as the triptan class is more clearly established. To some extent this conflict remains one of the great challenges for the next century.

The International Headache Society Committee on Clinical Trials in Migraine is currently recommending that the primary efficacy outcome should be headache-free at 2 hours. Although more rigid definitions have been recommended by the Committee for several years (The International Headache Society Clinical Trials Committee in Migraine 1991), the most commonly used definition for the primary endpoint has been the headache response or headache relief endpoint in which the patient treats an attack in the study only if they have a moderate or severe headache that is not improving. A patient is considered a responder if at 2 or 4 hours they have nil or mild headache (Goadsby *et al.* 1991). The sumatriptan clinical trial programme used this endpoint (Pilgrim 1991) and this has driven competitors to use similar outcome measures. Several issues arise, including the appropriate time (2 or 4 hours), the comparative value of the headache-free endpoint and the reporting of the outcomes from the trials.

**Table 7.1** Endpoints used in trials of acute migraine treatment

| Endpoint | At treatment* | Definition outcome* | Time |
| --- | --- | --- | --- |
| Headache response or relief | moderate/severe | nil/mild | 2 hr or 4 hr |
| Headache-free | moderate/severe | nil | 2 hr |
| Time-to-headache relief | moderate/severe | nil/mild | 0->2 hr |
| Meaningful headache relief | moderate/severe | patient defined | 2 hr |
| Complete response | moderate/severe | nil/mild + no recurrence** + no rescue medications† | 24 hr |
| Time-to *failure* | moderate/severe | patient takes rescue medication | 24 hr |

\* Headache severity after treatment with test substance at a defined time point
\*\* Recurrence: headache worsening to any level within 24 hr
† Within 24 hr

**Table 7.2** Clinical parameters used as endpoints

| Endpoint | Comment |
| --- | --- |
| Relief of pain | partial (nil or mild pain) compete (nil pain) |
| Relief of migraine-related symptoms | • nausea<br>• photophobia<br>• phonophobia |
| Relief of functional impairment | May be partial or complete |
| Time-to analysis | Survival curve methods |
| Consistency analysis | • placebo controlled<br>• open label |
| Tolerability | Non-serious adverse events |
| Absolute safety | • Biochemical/haematological tests<br>• Electrocardiography<br>• Serious adverse-event tracking |

## What fixed time points should be reported?

An issue independent to some extent from the endpoint used is when to make the measurement. There is an interaction between the need for convenience and the co-operation of subjects in a clinical trial, along with the need to obtain all relevant information. In terms of time one might argue that as soon as possible is, all other things being equal, the most useful outcome. This author takes the view that, for most patients with a moderately severe and certainly almost all patients with severe and disabling migraine, responses after 2 hours are generally unacceptable in high-end therapies. The natural history of a migraine attack is to terminate. Indeed how attacks terminate is one of the most interesting aspects of migraine pathophysiology in terms of understanding how to design better medicines (Goadsby 1997a). A recent study in which, by accident, all patients received placebo illustrates this concept beautifully (Figure 7.1). It can be seen that treatment with placebo results in a robust headache response of 37 per cent at 2 hours rising to 48 per cent at 4 hours (Jhee *et al.* 1998).

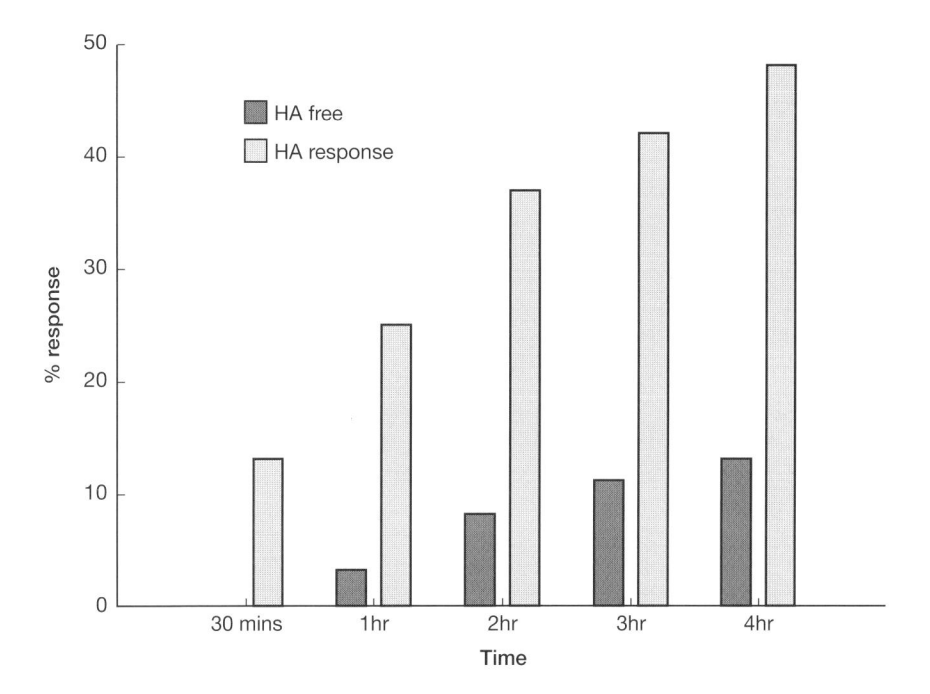

**Figure 7.1** Illustration of the time course of the placebo response in an acute migraine trial. From every time point, 30 minutes onwards, there is a placebo effect seen with the headache relief (moderate/severe pain becomes nil/mild) endpoint. There is a substantial penalty after two hours for collecting noise in the results. This effect is much less prominent when the headache-free endpoint is employed but no less valid, so that studies beyond four hours are inappropriate (Jhee *et al.* 1998)

The placebo effect is less of an issue with the headache-free endpoint. Considering these natural history data with population-based studies that show that patients place high value on rapid resolution of symptoms (Davies *et al.* 1998), it is very difficult to defend studies with endpoints beyond 2 hours and hard to understand why they would be reported for triptans.

*Survival study methods – time-to analysis*

In addition to considering which fixed time point is most appropriate, some recent comparative studies have been analysed using survival methodologies. These methods were used in the sumatriptan 100 mg versus oral cafergot study (The Multinational Oral Sumatriptan and Cafergot Study Group 1991) but not again until the rizatriptan development programme (Goadsby 1999). Literally, the analysis looks at how long headache survives from the time of initial treatment. These methods are widely used in other disciplines, such as oncology and multiple sclerosis (Prevention of Relapses and Disability by Interferon ß-1a Subcutaneously in Multiple Sclerosis Study Group 1998). The analysis applied in the rizatriptan studies (Tfelt-Hansen *et al.* 1998) is a variation on the Cox model methodology developed for discrete discontinuous data (Kalbfleisch & Prentice 1973). In effect the hazard ratio that is obtained gives the chance that one compound will reach the endpoint in question, here headache relief, sooner than another. The major advantage is that early time points of relief, which are valued highly by patients, are included in the analysis. Fixed time point methods discarding early time points are not clinically sensible, and may blur differences between treatments. The early time points allow a more robust comparison of the population treated, with the potential to detect modest differences. However, the method does not measure rates of response in terms of time so cannot lead to conclusions about speed of onset. This would be best done using stop-watch-type studies.

An example of the time to headache relief analysis would be the comparison between sumatriptan 100 mg and rizatriptan 10 mg (Tfelt-Hansen *et al.* 1998). The outcome was a hazard ratio of 1.21 (95% CI 1.02–1.44) demonstrating that over the 2-hour time period rizatriptan was more likely to produce headache relief in the next small period than sumatriptan.

## Headache response versus headache-free?

From the first suggestion that the major endpoint for migraine studies should not be complete pain relief there has been controversy. Certainly the International Headache Society Committee on Clinical Trials in Migraine (1991) incorporated headache-free in their initial recommendations, and recently decided to recommend headache-free at 2 hours as the primary endpoint in clinical trials (Tfelt-Hansen, personal communication).

Headache-free has a number of advantages: it is unambiguous and therefore does not require explanation, in contrast to headache response. Headache-free allows treatment of mild headache. In clinical practice patients will not necessarily wish to wait until they have moderate or severe headache to treat. The headache response construct demands this as the trigger to treatment, which is an artificial situation. Headache-free seems more sensitive to difference. As an example, the dose-response relationship for headache-free and headache relief for the zolmitriptan development programme are illustrated in Figure 7.2 (Goadsby 1998b). The differences between doses seem sharper at the lower end where one is trying to optimise the efficacy versus tolerability benefits of a compound.

The disadvantages of the headache-free endpoint include the view that for patients with slowly settling headache the transition to no pain is difficult to discern and for some patients the reduction in headache pain to mild is a substantial and very beneficial result. Cynically, it is said that the headache-free endpoint generates smaller percentage responses and this is less attractive to industry in terms of marketing. If headache-free can dissect the dose-response relationship, perhaps it would serve earlier phase studies better and more creative patient-focused endpoints might serve phase III studies better in terms of determining meaningful differences between new and established treatments.

## How to report studies?

Although it might be almost inappropriate to discuss this issue, it seems necessary to make some comments in this area. In the last decade the results of acute studies in migraine have been reported as point estimates, the proportion of patients reaching, for example, the headache response endpoint at 2 hours. An example of these data might be to report a 58 per cent response at 2 hours as the outcome from treatment with sumatriptan 100 mg (po). However, point estimates such as this provide no indication of the accuracy of the outcome. As an example, Tfelt-Hansen (1998) provides a meta-analysis of sumatriptan clinical trials and includes 95 per cent confidence interval calculations. The relevant calculations are shown in Table 7.3. It is essential that the results of studies are at least supplied with confidence intervals, although readers can estimate the 95 per cent confidence interval of a proportion relatively easily.

### *Confidence interval of the proportion p*

As an example, a patient takes a medication at time 0 in a randomised double-blind placebo-controlled study where patients may be randomised to placebo or active treatment arms. Two hours after taking the medication, they either have a response or do not. The population probability that they will have a response is $\pi$. In a particular study of $n$ patients, $r$ patients respond and therefore the proportion of responders is $p=r/n$.

An approximation to the 95 per cent confidence interval is:

$$95\%CIp = p \pm 1.96\sqrt{\frac{p(1-p)}{n}}$$

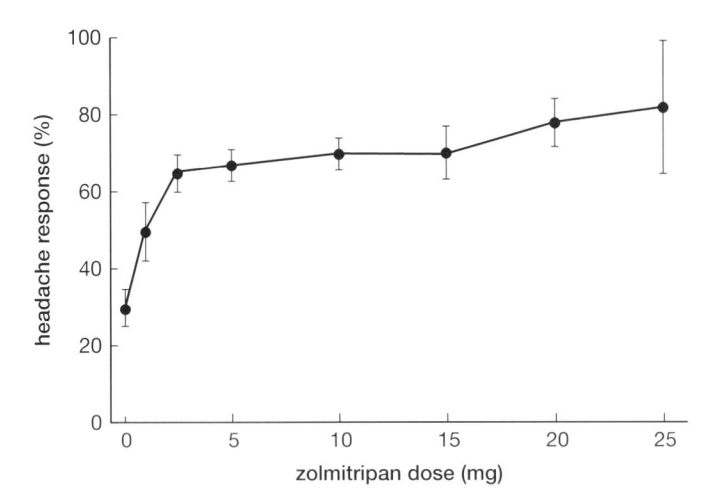

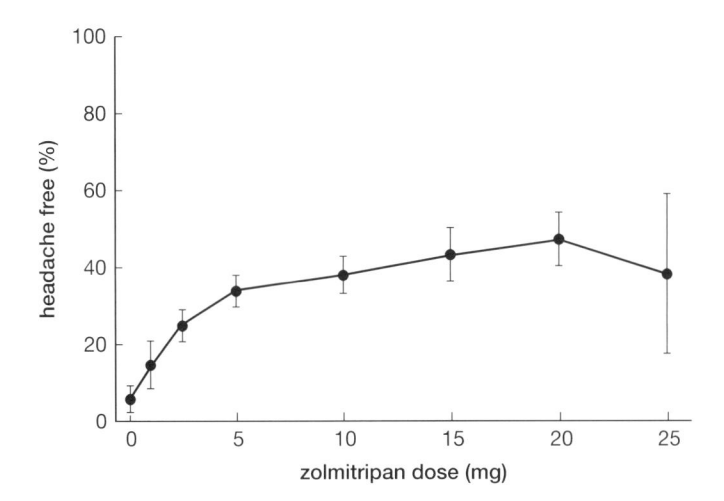

**Figure 7.2** Illustration of the dose-response relationship of zolmitriptan for headache relief (moderate/severe pain becomes nil/mild; Panel A) versus pain-free (Panel B) at two hours. The lower doses seem to separate better on the pain-free criterion and indeed this may help define the optimum dosing strategy

This is useful if $n$ is large and may be used particularly if $np>10$ and $n(1-p)>10$. The exact limits may be obtained from use of the $F$ distribution and the link between

**Table 7.3** An example of endpoint calculations

| Efficacy | Calculation | (%) | Response rate 95% confidence interval |
|---|---|---|---|
| placebo | 256/1036= | 25 | 22–28 |
| sumatriptan 100 mg | 1067/1854= | 58 | 56–60 |
| *Therapeutic gain* | | | |
| sumatriptan 100 mg | 58–25= | 33 | 30–36 |
| *NNT* | | | |
| sumatriptan 100 mg | 1/0.33= | 3.0 | 2.8–3.3 |

*Source*: Tfelt-Hansen (1998); see text for details of calculations

the $F$ and binomial distributions. For the interested reader the exact limits are (Armitage & Berry 1994):

$$95\% \ Lower = \frac{r}{r + (n - r + 1)F_{0.025, 2n - 2r + 2, 2r}}$$

$$95\% \ Upper = \frac{r}{r + 1 + (n - r)F^{-1}_{0.025, 2r + 2, 2n - 2r}}$$

## Particular endpoints of clinical interest?

Prescribers, payers and patients alike may have other endpoints that are of interest in a clinical trial. Most studies in acute migraine record information on the associated symptoms, such as nausea, photophobia and phonophobia, and give an indication of return to normal function. Associated symptoms almost without variation track the pain outcome and seldom add much to the pain analysis in terms of separating compounds. A possible exception is the data for early relief of nausea with rizatriptan (Tfelt-Hansen *et al.* 1998) which may be related to its relatively poor activity at the $5\text{-HT}_{1A}$ receptor (Goadsby 1998a), which in turn has some role in nausea generation (Grof *et al.* 1993; NewmanTancredi *et al.* 1998). Two issues, arguably of some importance, are consistency of response and side-effect potential.

### Consistency studies

Consistency in acute migraine studies may be derived from two sources, placebo-controlled blinded studies or open-label use. While open-label use mimics clinical practice and it is reassuring to know that a medicine that works will continue to work, this is somewhat self-fulfilling in these studies. Patients in these studies have had

## 84 Evidence and treatment

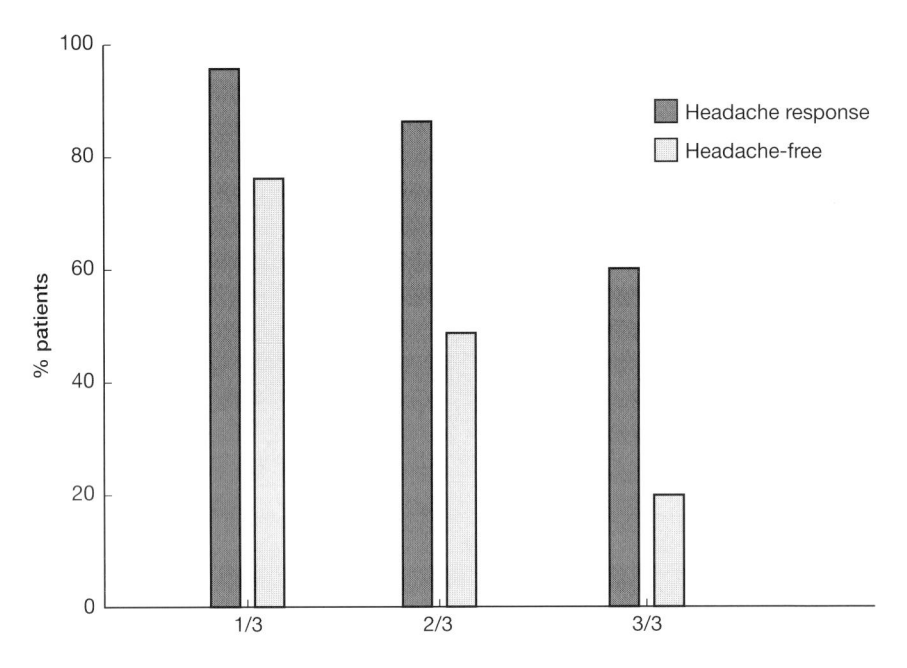

**Figure 7.3** Consistency of response of rizatriptan from a three-way double-blind placebo-controlled study reporting data for patients who completed the cross-over in the arms of the study that were placebo-controlled (*Source*: Kramer *et al.* 1998)

success in controlled studies and then keep taking medication for 6–12 months. Logically, most patients who stay in open-label studies will have good responses or they would drop out. It would be of interest to see more reporting of drop-out rates in these studies. To be able to compare consistency either head-to-head comparisons or relative comparisons from placebo-controlled trials are needed. Two well-controlled consistency studies have been published. The first, for sumatriptan 25 mg, 50 mg and 100 mg against placebo, shows that 61 per cent of patients responded in 2/3 attacks for sumatriptan 50 mg (Pfaffenrath *et al.* 1998). The second was completed in the rizatriptan development programme done as a three-way placebo-controlled cross-over study and shows that 86 per cent of patients responded in 2/3 attacks (Figure 7.3) (Kramer *et al.* 1998). Consistency is important to patients (Davies *et al.* 1998) and should form part of the overall assessment of any new compound.

### Adverse-event reporting

For some patients pain control comes at a considerable price in terms of side-effects and such patients place a great premium on a well-tolerated medication. One can use all causality adverse-event reporting as a crude measure of tolerability but not of safety (see below). By using them in this way the relative aggravation of any adverse event is not measured but this is offset in terms of utility by the large sample sizes running into thousands of patients for each of the triptan development programmes. It is a useful first approximation which does not seek to minimise side-effect variability or clinical significance. Adverse event rates can be used to perform dose selection trying to optimise efficacy against the side-effect price.

As an example, the selection of the 2.5 mg dose (Rapoport *et al.* 1997; Solomon *et al.* 1997) of zolmitriptan after initial strong development of the 5 mg dose (Dahlof *et al.* 1998) is a case in point. Figure 7.4 demonstrates the dose-response relationship for zolmitriptan across the development programme and the corresponding adverse-event rate. It can be seen that 2.5 mg, while on the shoulder of the efficacy-response relationship, lags behind 5 mg in terms of adverse events and thus represents a good balance for many patients. The naratriptan development programme developed this concept further by weighting dose selection for tolerability more strongly than for efficacy (Goadsby 1997b). The outcome is, in general terms, the best tolerated of the currently available triptans.

### Safety

All the triptans currently used (sumatriptan, naratriptan, rizatriptan and zolmitriptan), and those in late development (eletriptan, almotriptan and frovatriptan) are $5\text{-HT}_{1B}$ agonists (Goadsby 1998a) and thus constrict human coronary vessels to some degree (MaassenVanDenBrink *et al.* 1998). All seem relatively safe but none is safer than the others. Some are better tolerated, and this applies most clearly to naratriptan, but this must not be confused with cardiovascular safety, which is identical across the class.

## Therapeutic gain and number needed to treat

There has been some interest in recent times in summary measures that try to express the overall utility of a medication and perhaps more so for new medications where cost-benefit considerations are becoming more important. In terms of comparing new medicines, a randomised controlled clinical trial remains the gold standard for comparing drugs. However, these trials do not exist for all the currently used acute migraine treatments and so some summary measures, such as the therapeutic gain and the number needed to treat (NNT), provide first approximations of the general response of a compound (Goadsby 1998b).

### Therapeutic gain

This is the simple calculation of subtracting the placebo response from a randomised trial away from the active response to try to estimate how much of the effect seen is due to the compound. For any comparison of therapeutic gains there is an assumption that the effects of placebo are additive, and this is not at all clear. There is also a ceiling effect that works against the calculation to minimise differences in that one almost never sees a 100 per cent headache response rate and

**A**

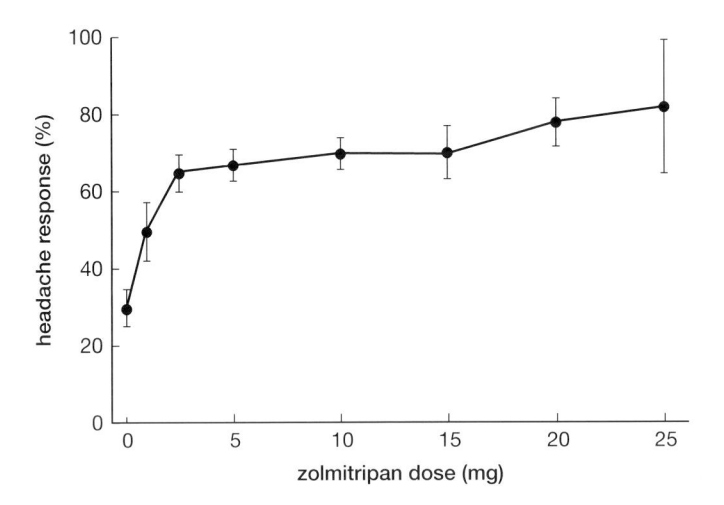

**B**

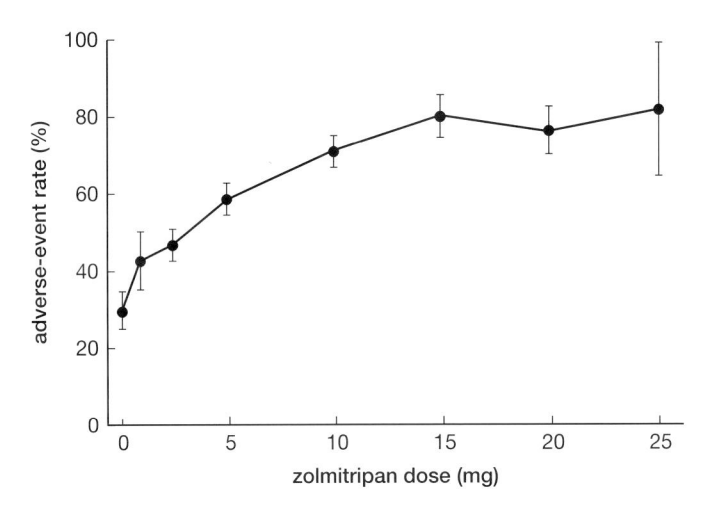

**Figure 7.4** Illustration of the dose-response relationship for efficacy (Panel A) and adverse events (Panel B) for the zolmitriptan development programme. The 2.5 mg dose being selected to combine good efficacy with reasonable tolerability

indeed not much more than 80 per cent for oral triptan studies, but the placebo responses vary between 15 and 45 per cent, thus telescoping to some extent the outcome of therapeutic gain calculations. This is less of an issue if one does a meta-analysis across large numbers of patients since the placebo responses are reasonably consistent.

Across the naratriptan, rizatriptan and zolmitriptan development programmes for the headache response endpoint for which there are the most data, the placebo responses were 27 per cent (95% CI 24–30 per cent), 37 per cent (33–41 per cent) and 29 per cent (24–34 per cent), respectively. This compares with 24 per cent (21–27 per cent) for the published meta-analysis of the sumatriptan studies (Tfelt-Hansen 1998). It should be remarked that confidence intervals for the differences between a proportion can be calculated and a typical calculation is listed in Table 7.3, on p.83. If one wished to know the difference in the response between the placebo ($p$) and the active treatment ($a$), therapeutic gain, $p-a$, confidence interval for that difference would be (Armitage & Berry 1994):

$$95\% \; CI \; (p - a) = (p - a) \pm 1.96 \sqrt{\frac{p(1-p)}{n} + \frac{a(1-a)}{m}}$$

A comparison of the 2-hour headache response rates for sumatriptan, naratriptan 2.5 mg, rizatriptan 10 mg and zolmitriptan 2.5 mg is shown in Figure 7.5 and illustrates the potential benefit of the therapeutic gain calculation in terms of correcting for placebo effects. It remains true in clinical practice that the triptans are different and thus Figure 7.5 illustrates the crude nature of these types of comparisons which fail to reveal differences that will be reported in clinic.

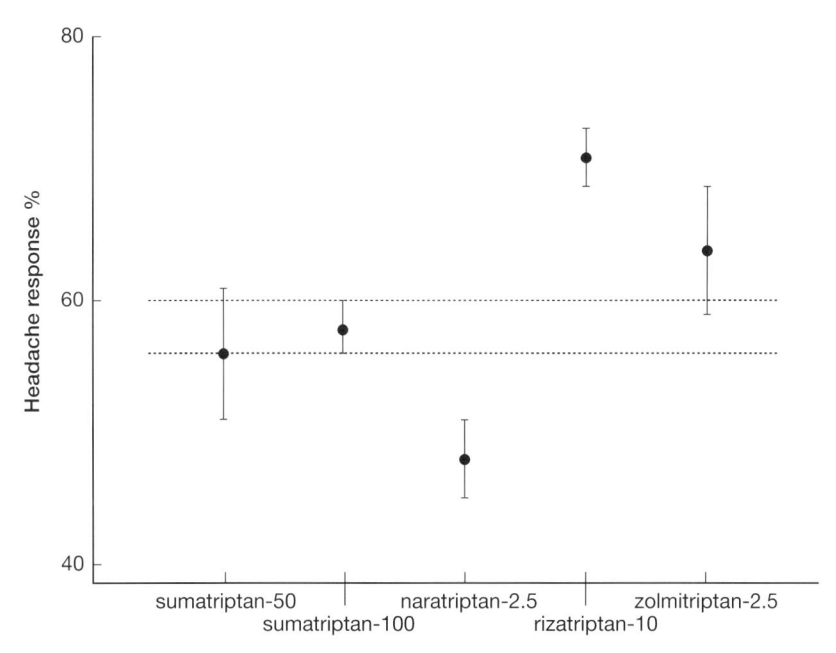

**Figure 7.5** *(cont.)*

**B**

[Chart showing therapeutic gain % for sumatriptan-50, sumatriptan-100, naratriptan-2.5, rizatriptan-10, and zolmitriptan-2.5, with data points around 73% for most, and ~61% for naratriptan-2.5]

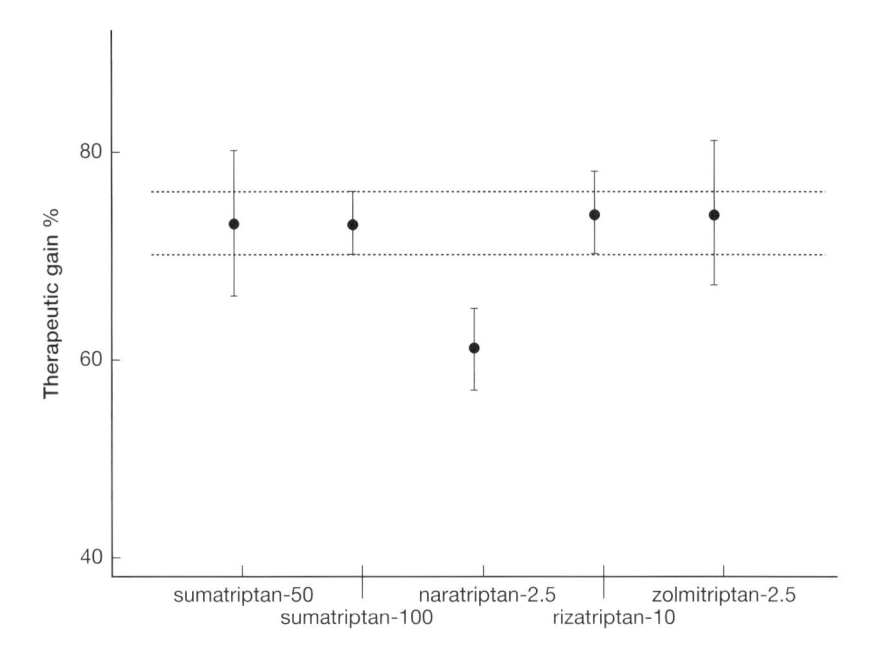

**Figure 7.5** Comparison of headache response rates for doses of triptans used in clinical practice. In Panel A the uncorrected headache response is shown and in Panel B the therapeutic gains. It is clear from the perspective of therapeutic gain calculations that sumatriptan, rizatriptan and zolmitriptan are very similar at 2 hours, with only naratriptan performing consistently less well. The latter outcome is in line with direct comparator studies. Each data point is presented with the 95 per cent confidence interval and the dashed line is for reference to sumatriptan 100 mg

## Number needed to treat

The NNT is the reciprocal of the difference between the response on active medication and that on placebo taken as a proportion. It is no more than the inverse of the therapeutic gain when expressed as a proportion. The calculation for sumatriptan is illustrated in Table 7.3, on p.83. Similarly, adverse-event rates can be summarised by subtracting the placebo to derive a number needed to harm (NNH). This is an unfortunate term since most adverse events in acute migraine trials are mild and transient and certainly do no harm. However, the use of the term is not a big issue unless it is inadequately explained. All the problems that were outlined above apply to NNT calculations, especially the limitations. A particular danger with NNT calculations is to see them expressed without confidence intervals as though the one number summarised what is known about the compound. The folly of this is illustrated in Figure 7.6. NNTs are point estimates and as such they have error. Moreover, the error can be large and important when it overlaps for two compounds

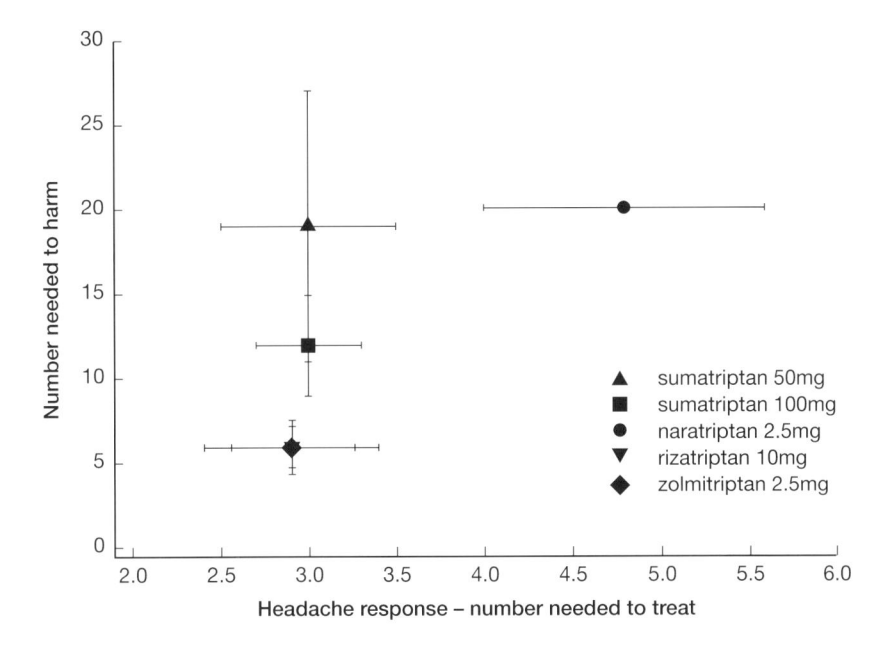

**Figure 7.6** Comparison of number needed to treat (NNT) and number needed to harm (NNH) for the triptans. This analysis suggests they are very similar in both dimensions with only naratriptan being demonstrably different. There is no confidence interval for naratriptan adverse events (NNH) because the difference is so small from placebo rendering the calculations less useful

and suggests there may actually be no difference between them. NNT calculations have been used as crude measures of cost per effective treatment by multiplying by the dose cost but again, without confidence intervals, this calculation is almost completely meaningless and indeed may be deceptive.

## Conclusions

The study of migraine in clinical trials has come a long way in the last decade with the standardisation of patient groups and some very considerable similarities in entry and endpoint measurements across development programmes for new medicines. Unfortunately, the endpoints we use are somewhat crude. Migraine is much more than headache so that by measuring headache relief as an endpoint there is much about the new treatments that is not captured. The challenge for the future is to understand the benefits, and the disadvantages, of the current treatments from the patient's perspective so that we can tease out important differences between treatments and thus design studies and ultimately make evidence-based decisions when selecting treatments for acute migraine.

## Acknowledgements

The author is a Wellcome Senior Research Fellow. The work reviewed in this chapter has been supported by the Wellcome Trust and the Migraine Trust.

## References

Armitage P & Berry G (1994). *Statistical methods in medical research* 3rd edn. Blackwell Science, Oxford.

Davies GM, Santanello NC, Kramer M, Matzura-Wolfe D & Lipton RB (1998). Determinants of patient satisfaction with migraine treatment. *Headache* **38**, 380.

Dahlof C, Diener HC, Goadsby PJ et al. (1998). Zolmitriptan, a $5HT_{1B/1D}$ receptor agonist for the acute oral treatment of migraine: a multicentre, dose-range finding study. *European Journal of Neurology* **5**, 535–43.

Goadsby PJ (1997a). Current concepts of the pathophysiology of migraine. In *Neurologic clinics of North America* Vol.15 (ed. NT Mathew), pp.27–41. WB Saunders, Philadelphia.

Goadsby PJ (1997b). Naratriptan in the treatment of acute migraine attacks. *Prescriber* **8**, 89–97.

Goadsby PJ (1998a). $5HT_{1B/1D}$ agonists in migraine: comparative pharmacology and its therapeutic implications. *CNS Drugs* **10**, 271–86.

Goadsby PJ (1998b). A triptan too far. *J Neurol Neurosurg Psychiatry* **64**, 143–7.

Goadsby PJ (1999). Rizatriptan in the treatment of acute migraine attacks. *Prescriber* **10** (in press).

Goadsby PJ, Zagami AS, Donnan GA et al. (1991). A double blind placebo controlled crossover study of sumatriptan in the treatment of acute migraine attacks. *Lancet* **338**, 782–3.

Grof P, Joffe R, Kennedy S, Persad E, Syrotiuk J & Bradford D (1993). An open study of oral flesinoxan, a 5-Ht(1a) receptor agonist, in treatment-resistant depression. *International Clinical Psychopharmacology* **8**(3), 167–72.

The International Headache Society Committee on Clinical Trials in Migraine (1991). Guidelines for controlled trials of drugs in migraine. *Cephalalgia* **11**, 1–12.

Jhee SS, Salazar DE, Ford NF, Fulmor IE, Sramek JJ & Cutler NR (1998). Monitoring of acute migraine attacks: placebo response and safety data. *Headache* **38**, 35–8.

Kalbfleisch JD & Prentice RL (1973). Marginal likelihoods based on Cox's regression and life model. *Biometrika* **60**, 267–78.

Kramer MS, Matzura-Wolfe D, Polis A et al. (1998). A placebo-controlled crossover study of rizatriptan in the treatment of multiple migraine attacks. *Neurology* **51**, 773–81.

Lance JW & Goadsby PJ (1998). *Mechanism and management of headache* 6th edn. Butterworth-Heinemann, London.

MaassenVanDenBrink A, Reekers M, Bax WA, Ferrari MD & Saxena PR (1998). Coronary side-effect potential of current and prospective antimigraine drugs. *Circulation* **98**, 25–30.

The Multinational Oral Sumatriptan and Cafergot Study Group (1991). A randomized, double-blind comparison of sumatriptan and cafergot in the acute treatment of migraine. *Eur Neurol* **31**, 314–22.

NewmanTancredi A, Gavaudan S, Conte C et al. (1998). Agonist and antagonist actions of antipsychotic agents at $5-HT_{1A}$ receptors: a [S-35]GTP gamma S binding study. *Eur J Pharmacol* **355**(2–3), 245–56.

Pfaffenrath V, Cunin G, Sjonell G & Prendergast S (1998). Efficacy and safety of sumatriptan tablets (25 mg, 50 mg, and 100 mg) in the acute treatment of migraine; defining the optimum doses of oral sumatriptan. *Headache* **38**, 184–90.

Pilgrim AJ (1991). Methodology of clinical trials of sumatriptan in migraine and cluster headache. *Eur Neurol* **31**, 295–9.

Prevention of Relapses and Disability by Interferon β-1a Subcutaneously in Multiple Sclerosis Study Group (1998). Randomised double-blind placebo-controlled study of interferon ß-1a in relapsing/remitting multiple sclerosis. *Lancet* **352**, 1498–504.

Rapoport AM, Ramadan NM, Adelman JU *et al.* (1997). Optimizing the dose of zolmitriptan (Zomig, 311C90) for the acute treatment of migraine. *Neurology* **49**, 1210–18.

Solomon GD, Cady RK, Klapper JA, Earl NL, Saper JR & Ramadan NM (1997). Clinical efficacy and tolerability of 2.5mg zolmitriptan for the acute treatment of migraine. *Neurology* **49**, 1219–25.

Tfelt-Hansen P (1998). Efficacy and adverse events of subcutaneous, oral, and intranasal sumatriptan used for migraine treatment: a systematic review based on number needed to treat. *Cephalalgia* **18**, 538.

Tfelt-Hansen P, Teall J, Rodriguez F *et al.* (1998). Oral rizatriptan versus oral sumatriptan: a direct comparative study in the acute treatment of migraine. *Headache* **38**, 748–55.

Chapter 8

# Cost-effectiveness of migraine therapy: evaluating new acute treatments

*David Millson, Harry Ward, Wendy Clark and Martin Frischer*

## Introduction

Migraine is a chronic, episodic condition in which patients experience headaches with varying degrees of severity and associated disability. Migraine is common, with around 10–12 per cent of the general population classified as 'active migraineurs', having had at least one attack within the previous 12 months (Lipton *et al.* 1998). In these patients, median attack frequency is 1.5 per month and duration under one day, although at least 10 per cent of patients have weekly attacks and in one-fifth the attacks last 2–3 days (Ferrari 1998b).

Migraine has highest prevalence during the period of life of greatest economic productivity (Solomon & Price 1997) with consequent significant impact on the financial burden to society. This comprises both direct costs, to the health care provider (e.g. pharmaceutical and dispensing costs, physician consultations and different forms of hospital contact), and indirect costs, which include the economic costs to society owing to absence from, and impaired productivity at work.

This chapter presents an economic evaluation relating to the acute treatment of migraine with oral prescription therapy, comparing the available published data with regard to the triptans to those of conventional migraine therapy. It analyses current use of health care resources as captured by general practice research database (GPRD) data (Rodríguez & Gutthann 1998) and prescription analysis and cost (PACT) data (Frischer & Chapman 1998), together with a critical appraisal of published economic and clinical data, limited to randomised controlled trials. Over-the-counter medication is not considered. Cost-effectiveness is also assessed, from both a health care provider's and societal perspective.

## Methods

A systematic search of the literature was conducted for peer-reviewed papers referring to health economic assessments for the triptans. All current triptan manufacturers were approached for further relevant unpublished information. PACT data for the West Midlands, representing around 5.5 million people (10 per cent of the population of England) were searched for by British National Formulary (BNF) categories related to the acute treatment of migraine. Prescribing data for each quarter are presented. The GPRD, which holds data on a representative cumulative sample (5–10 per cent) of patients in the West Midlands, was searched for migraine diagnosis, treatment and referral data.

## 94 Evidence and treatment

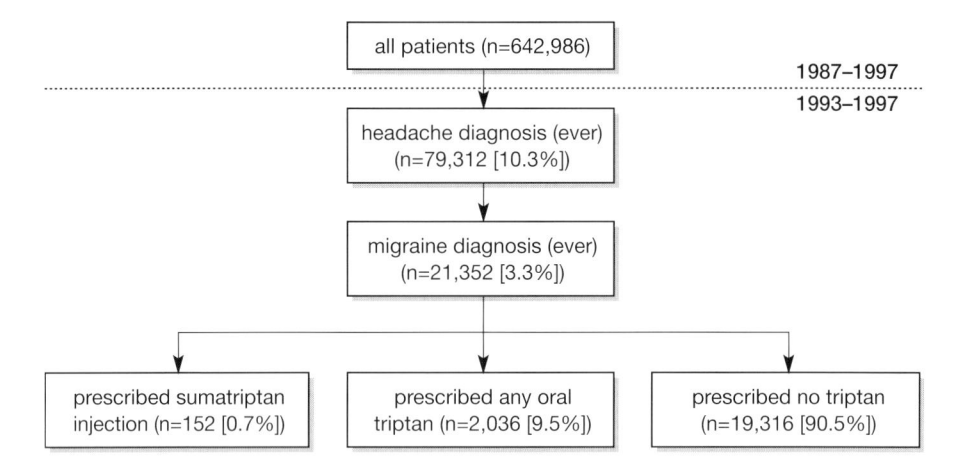

```
all patients (n=642,986)
        │
        │  ┄┄┄┄┄┄┄┄┄  1987–1997
        ▼              1993–1997
headache diagnosis (ever)
   (n=79,312 [10.3%])
        │
        ▼
migraine diagnosis (ever)
   (n=21,352 [3.3%])
   ┌────┼────┐
   ▼    ▼    ▼
```

| prescribed sumatriptan injection (n=152 [0.7%]) | prescribed any oral triptan (n=2,036 [9.5%]) | prescribed no triptan (n=19,316 [90.5%]) |

**Figure 8.1** Cumulative GPRD data (1993–7) for headache & migraine diagnosis and triptan prescriptions

Much higher use of emergency room and specialist consultations for migraine in North America makes extrapolation of direct treatment costs to Europe and the UK difficult (Ferrari 1998a) Therefore, this paper will confine itself to drawing general inferences from non-European literature. Each of the critical factors contributing to the assessment of cost-benefit will be reviewed independently.

## How many UK patients currently have a diagnosis of migraine according to primary care records?

The GPRD holds individual patient diagnostic and prescription records together with hospital contacts. Participating general practitioners are required to record every prescription and all significant morbidity and consultation items (Rodríguez & Gutthann 1998). The GPRD was used to conduct a preliminary analysis of the diagnosis of headache, migraine and use of sumatriptan injection, oral triptans or conventional therapy over a 5-year period (1993–7). Out of a sample of 642,986 individual patient records more than 10 per cent had a diagnosis of headache, and around 3 per cent had a specific diagnosis of migraine (Figure 8.1).

The diagnosis rates reported from the GPRD are consistent with those reported in other recent primary care surveys (3–10 per cent) in the UK (Dr Bill Holmes & Dr Bill Laughey, personal communication) but considerably lower than the 12 per cent migraine prevalence figure reported by Lipton *et al.* (1998) using a UK random telephone-based survey using IHS diagnostic criteria.

## Have the triptans demonstrated improved efficacy ...

The principal efficacy endpoint chosen from clinical trials for use in the economic analysis was the 2-hour headache response rate, i.e. the proportion of patients whose headache severity improved to mild or no pain on a 4-point scale within two hours of treatment. Recurrence rate, the proportion of responders in whom headache returned within 24–48 hours, was also considered in some studies.

### (a) ... compared to conventional therapy?

The triptans are generally considered to be more effective than oral ergotamine plus caffeine or aspirin plus metoclopramide preparations. However, there are no fully published reports of good-quality randomised placebo-controlled studies comparing the new-generation triptans to conventional therapy. The results from a single-blind study comparing rizatriptan to standard care (predominantly sumatriptan) are available only in abstract form (Block *et al.* 1998). This study represents an extension of the double-blind phase III trials. Such a design has increased potential for bias.

Well-designed controlled trials with oral sumatriptan versus conventional therapy – aspirin/metoclopramide, cafergot & tolfenamic acid – have been published in full (Table 8.1).

Two published studies compared oral sumatriptan 100 mg with a high-dose aspirin/metoclopramide combination (900 mg/10 mg). One study considered efficacy over two attacks of migraine, demonstrating no statistically significant differences between the two treatment groups in primary or secondary efficacy variables (Tfelt-Hansen *et al.* 1995). The second study evaluated efficacy over three migraine attacks and reported a significantly more rapid and greater relief of headache symptoms with sumatriptan. However, sumatriptan therapy was associated

**Table 8.1** Comparative efficacy of migraine therapies

| Paired comparison | No. of studies | No. of patients | Response rate difference (95%) CI |
|---|---|---|---|
| Oral sumatriptan versus ergotamine/caffeine | 1 | 577 | 17.9% (9.1–26.8%) |
| Oral sumatriptan versus acetylsalicylic acid plus metoclopramide | 2 | 610 | 12.3% (–4.5–+29%) Not statistically significant |
| Oral sumatriptan versus tolfenamic acid | 1 | 141 | –2% (–17–+21%) Not statistically significant |

*Sources:* Canadian Co-ordinating Office for Health Technology Assessment (1997); Myllylä *et al.* (1998)

with higher recurrence (The Oral Sumatriptan and Aspirin plus Metoclopramide Comparative Study Group 1992) and impaired tolerability (Tfelt-Hansen *et al.* 1995). In a direct comparison with Cafergot (oral ergotamine 2 mg and caffeine 200 mg), sumatriptan 100 mg was consistently significantly more effective at reducing the intensity of the headache at two hours and provided more rapid relief. Cafergot was, however, associated with lower recurrence at 48 hours (The Multinational Oral Sumatriptan and Cafergot Comparative Study Group 1992).

More recently, the results from a double-blind placebo-controlled comparative study of sumatriptan 100 mg tablets versus rapid-release tolfenamic acid tablets 200 mg have been published. Over two migraine attacks the two active drugs were significantly more effective than placebo at reducing the intensity of the headache at two hours, with no significant difference between the two active treatments. There were no significant differences in headache recurrence between the three treatment arms (Myllylä *et al.* 1998).

### (b) ... compared to oral sumatriptan?

Both Goadsby (1998) and Ferrari (1998b) have recently reviewed comparative 2-hour headache response data and therapeutic benefit from placebo-controlled trials conducted with the triptans. Goadsby only considered sumatriptan, naratriptan and zolmitriptan. Whereas Ferrari also considered the recently launched rizatriptan and concluded, 'At this time, only tentative conclusions can be drawn from comparisons with oral sumatriptan.' Considering the attributes claimed for each triptan, Ferrari states that 'Naratriptan 2.5 mg has a slower onset of action with slightly lower response rates, but shows slightly less headache recurrence and is tolerated better. Zolmitriptan 2.5–5.0 mg is well tolerated, is at least as effective, and may show improved within-patient consistency. Rizatriptan 10 mg has slightly higher response rates and probably a better within-patient consistency, while tolerability is similar ...'

To identify true clinical differences comparator trials over multiple attacks are needed. This is supported by a meta-analysis of published triptan trials by Tepper & Millson (1998) showing that calculated number of patients needed to treat (NNT) to

**Table 8.2** Cost of migraine treatments in the UK at the doses used in comparative trials

| Drug | Dose | Cost (£)* |
| --- | --- | --- |
| Sumatriptan | 100 mg | 8.00 |
| Aspirin/metoclopramide | 900 mg/10 mg | 0.33 |
| Ergotamine/caffeine | 2 mg/200 mg | 0.39 |
| Tolfenamic acid rapid release | 200 mg | 1.50 |

\* *Prices from December 1998 MIMS & September 1998 BNF*

## Cost-effectiveness of migraine therapy 97

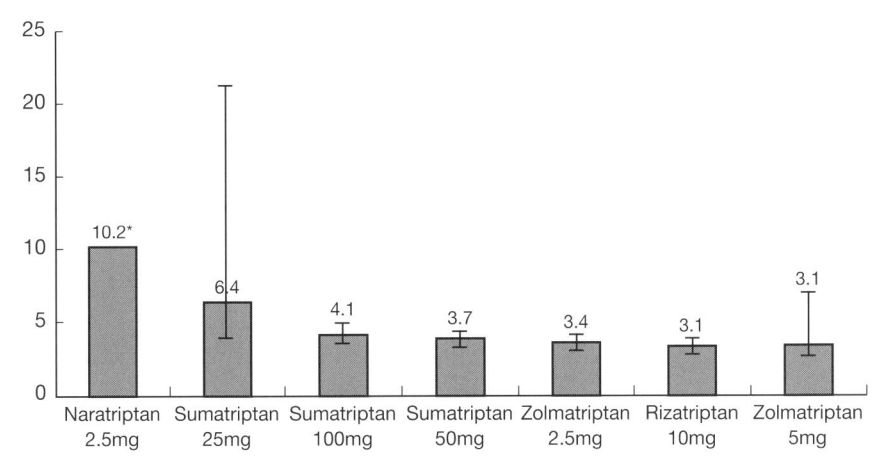

* Results from the trial meeting the specified selection criteria were non-significant, producing a lower 95 per cent CI of 4.6 and an infinite upper interval. The inclusion of a crossover trial (Mathew et al. 1997) estimates NNT (95%CI) to be 6.1 (3.9, 14.6). The reader should note that this NNT calculation is derived from a single study. Goadsby (p.89), using all available data from the phase II/III studies, estimates the NNT for naratriptan as 4.8.
CI = confidence interval; NNT = number of patients needed to be treated to obtain a 2-hour headache response attributable to treatment

**Figure 8.2** NNT values for triptans (lower number indicates higher efficacy). Error Bars Indicate 95% CIs (*Source*: Tepper & Millson 1998)

demonstrate a benefit over placebo was between 2.0 and 4.0 for all the triptans (with the exception of naratriptan >6.0) (see Figure 8.2). Whereas the comparable NNT for high-dose aspirin metoclopramide reported by the Oxford Evidence Based Medicine Group was 3.1 (Anon 1996). To date, all of the new triptans have reported either improved 2-hour efficacy with the exception of naratriptan (Visser *et al.* 1996; Tepper 1998; Tfelt-Hansen *et al.* 1998) or lower recurrence with the exception of rizatriptan relative to oral sumatriptan (Goadsby 1998).

## How many and which types of migraine treatment are prescribed in the UK?

Aggregated PACT data for all the 13 health authorities in the West Midlands are presented to give an overview of the different migraine treatments prescribed between June 1993 and June 1998 (Figure 8.3). Prescribing volume over this five-year period rose from just under 850,000 to around 1,200,000 unit doses per quarter. The first 5-HT$_1$ agonist, sumatriptan, (launched in 1991/2) gradually increased its market share from around 30,000 to 110,000 unit doses per quarter, while the volume of other antimigraine drugs (including analgesic/anti-emetic combinations, ergotamine preparations and isometheptene) remained relatively unchanged. The first of the new

**Drugs for treatment of acute migraine attacks**

[Chart: Log Unit Doses/Quarter from Jun-93 to Jun-98]

Legend:
— Analgesics with Anti-Emetics
—·— Antimigraine Drug 1
— — Antimigraine Drug 2
▬▬ NSAID 1
········ 5-HT$_1$ Agonist 1
—··— 5-HT$_1$ Agonist 2
▬▬ 5-HT$_1$ Agonist 3
------ All Migraine Treatments

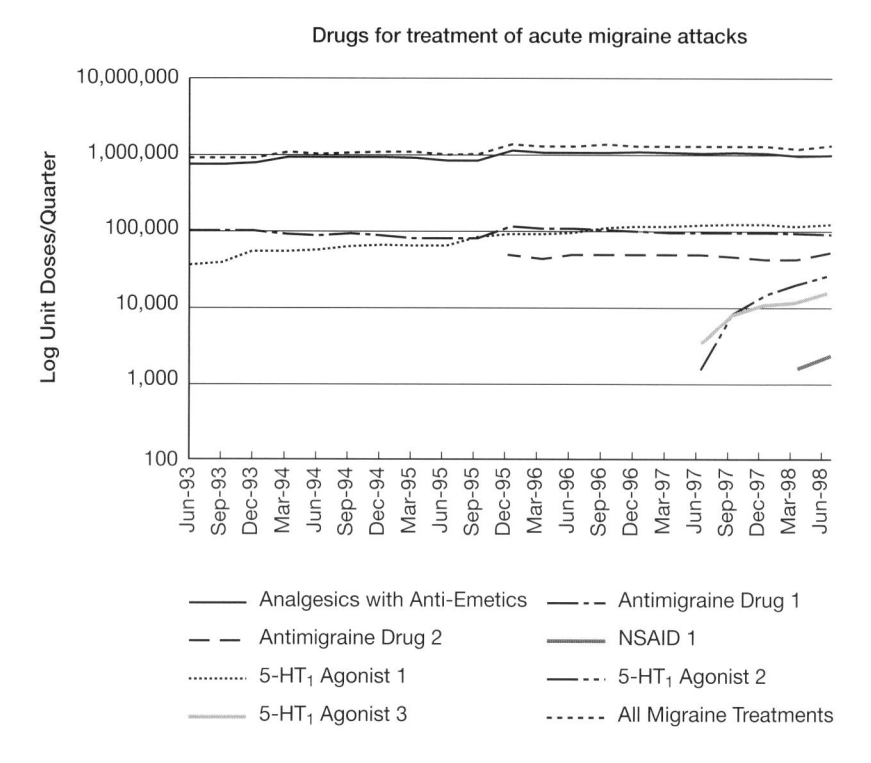

**Figure 8.3** West Midlands PACT data analysis: unit doses of drugs prescribed for the treatment of migraine, in primary care, 1993–1998

entrant triptans, introduced in early 1997, have shown a steady increase in prescribing volume. The GPRD analysis indicates that approximately 10 per cent of migraine patients (who were prescribed medication) received treatment with a triptan (9.5 per cent oral, 0.5 per cent injection) over the period 1993–7 (see Figure 8.1, on p.94).

## How does the cost of treating a migraine attack compare across the triptans?

While total aggregated prescribing volume for all migraine treatments has risen by 40 per cent over the last five years, the associated drug costs have increased by nearly 200 per cent, from around £380,000 to £1,120,000 per quarter. The vast majority of this additional expenditure was due to the triptans, which accounted for 66 per cent of migraine drug costs in 1993, increasing to 85 per cent in 1998.

Recent UK promotional material has suggested large cost differentials between the triptans, with costs per attack ranging from £8.00 for naratriptan to £28.00 for sumatriptan. This analysis is based on the maximum 'safe dose' which can be given

Cost-effectiveness of migraine therapy 99

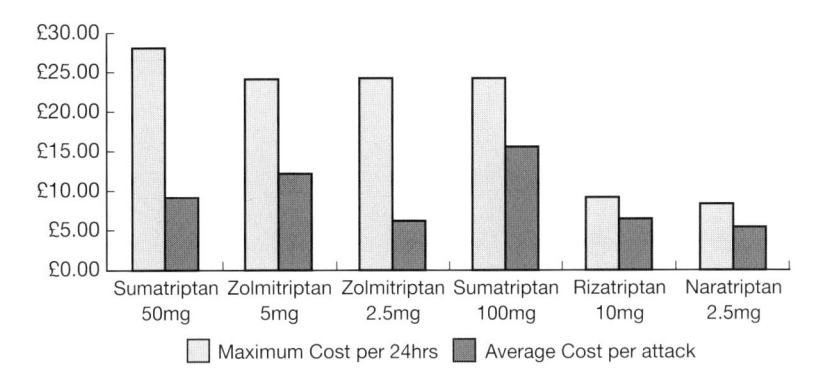

**Figure 8.4** Cost comparison chart of oral 5-HT$_1$ agonists – maximum 'safe dose' in 24hrs versus mean number of tablets per attack

in a 24-hour period, as described in the summary of product characteristics (see lighter bars in Figure 8.4). This is a maximum tolerated dose based on an assessment of the safety margin for a product, and is a reflection of the therapeutic index or risk:benefit (European Commission 1998). A more meaningful comparison between the triptans would relate to the WHO defined daily dose or the mean number of tablets used to treat an attack. When recalculated based on this more clinically relevant parameter, then the cost of all triptans falls largely within the range of £5.00–10.00 per attack (see darker bars in Figure 8.4).

## Does triptan therapy reduce associated direct health care costs?

A number of health economic models used in pharmaceutical marketing assume reduced hospital contact for patients treated with triptan therapy compared with conventional treatment. This assumption may be appropriate in a managed care system, such as in the USA, where there is high emergency room use (Ferrari 1998a). However, UK-specific data on migraine-related hospital contacts demonstrate a 6–12-fold increase particularly in outpatient referral rates for patients receiving triptans. Hospital contact rates were particularly high for patients receiving injectable sumatriptan (546/1,000), were less than half this for patients receiving oral triptans (213/1,000) and less than one-tenth of this for patients receiving conventional or 'usual' therapy (46/1,000) (see Figure 8.1 and Table 8.3). The reasons for these large differences are currently unknown and require further explanation. They may reflect the greater migraine disability of those patients being referred, opinion leader-led prescribing, primary care physicians seeking confirmation of the diagnosis and/or an endorsement by secondary care specialists before prescribing a more specific and

**Table 8.3** All hospital migraine specific contacts for migraine 1993–7 derived from West Midlands GPRD data

| Hospital contact | Migraine – no triptan (n=19,316) No. (%) | Cost (£) | Migraine + oral triptans (n= 2,036) No. (%) | Cost (£) | Migraine + injectable sumatriptan (n=152) No. (%) | Cost (£) |
|---|---|---|---|---|---|---|
| Referral to A&E | 64 (0.33) | 2,368 | 30 (1.47) | 1,110 | 5 (3.29) | 185 |
| Inpatient hospital discharge | 79 (0.41) | 85,162 | 27 (1.33) | 29,106 | 6 (3.95) | 6,468 |
| Outpatient referral | 727 (3.7) | 45,801 | 364 (17.88) | 22,932 | 65 (42.76) | 4,095 |
| Inpatient hospital admission | 22 (0.11) | NC | 13 (0.64) | NC | 7 (4.6) | NC |
| All hospital contacts | 892 (4.62) | £133,331 | 434 (21.32) | £53,148 | 83 (54.6) | £10,748 |
| Rate per 1,000 patients | 46 | £6,903 | 213 | £26,104 | 546 | £70,710 |

NC = Not costed length of stay unknown

more expensive therapy. Such increased hospital consultations alone may increase differential costs over 'usual care' of nearly £20.00 per patient per year.

## Are the triptan cost-effective treatments for migraine?

Economic evaluation as described by Drummond *et al.* (1997) addresses the issue of choice between different therapies, including in some circumstances the 'do nothing' alternative (i.e. placebo in randomised controlled trials). It analyses the costs and consequences of each option in order to inform the decision maker(s). There are three main types of economic evaluation:

- *cost-effectiveness analysis* compares therapies whose outcome can be measured in the same units, for example, cost per life years gained. Therefore this type of analysis may not address all the outcomes associated with an intervention.

- *cost-benefit analysis* seeks to measure all the costs and benefits associated with a particular therapy compared with a 'do nothing' option. In order to carry out the analysis the benefits of the therapy (e.g. relief of pain and suffering) are converted to monetary values. This type of analysis provides information on the absolute benefit of the programme, as it measures costs and benefits in the same terms.

- *cost-utility analysis* seeks to measure outcomes in terms of quality-adjusted life years, a generic measure of the value of the intervention. This enables programmes with different outcomes to be compared without the need to express the benefits in monetary terms.

In this chapter we employ the technique of cost-effectiveness analysis, as we are seeking to compare the triptans with the conventional treatment employed in the UK of aspirin plus metoclopramide preparations. The analysis is carried out from two perspectives: the National Health Service and society as a whole. The results of this analysis using sumatriptan as an example are shown below.

## Cost-effectiveness from an NHS perspective

The analysis in Table 8.4 relates to drug cost only: there may be other NHS costs/savings. Extrapolation from GPRD data suggests that patients receiving triptans make more extensive use of secondary services than those prescribed other treatments. However, there is no confirmatory evidence to substantiate changing NHS costs in either a positive or negative direction. In order to confirm these effects, prospective data on the use of NHS services would need to be collected as part of a randomised controlled trial comparing the triptans against aspirin/metoclopramide.

**Table 8.4** Drug cost per migraine aborted per year (based on median of 18 attacks per year)

| Treatment strategy | Drug cost for 1 year (£) | Expected efficacy (%) | Incremental cost (£) | Additional attacks aborted | Cost per additional aborted attack (£) |
|---|---|---|---|---|---|
| ASA/Meto | 5.76 | 44 | | | |
| Oral Sum | 144 | 56 | 138.24 | 2.16 | 64.00 |

*Sources:* Canadian Co-ordinating Office for Health Technology Assessment (1997); Ferrari (1998b)

## Cost-effectiveness from a societal perspective

The average number of working days lost to migraine ranges from 6.75 to 12.6 per year in the models presented by the pharmaceutical industry (Daly & Hurst 1998; Wells 1998; Dr Chris Allen, personal communication). Triptan treatment has been demonstrated to reduce the number of working days lost to migraine, compared to 'usual care', by 35–54 per cent (Gross *et al.* 1996; Mushey *et al.* 1996; Daly & Hurst 1998). Thus, the potential economic benefit to society using £18,215 as the average UK yearly income (ILO) is £187–539 per person per year.

With consideration of the incremental direct drug costs (Table 8.4), the above analysis suggests that there is a net economic gain to society of £49–401 per person per year with triptan therapy. If the increased use of hospital resources, as identified by GPRD, is included, the net economic gain to society lies between £29–381 per patient per year.

## Cost-utility analysis

No published cost-utility analyses exist for the UK for the treatment of migraine using the triptans. The Canadian Co-ordinating Office for Health Technology Assessment (1997) has published an independent cost-utility analysis and these data have been quoted (see Table 8.5).

In the absence of a UK-derived utility analysis these Canadian data may give decision makers further insight into the issues. As a benchmark the Development and Evaluation Committee (DEC) considers that a cost utility of less than £20,000 per life year supported by high-quality clinical evidence provides a strong recommendation for the use of a product (Stevens *et al.* 1995).

## Should the NHS fund triptan therapy?

NHS-funded triptan use poses a dilemma. While efficacy benefits with the triptans are likely in some patients, all costs are borne by the NHS, yet the potential benefits are likely to be societal gains.

**Table 8.5** Cost-utility analysis

| | Cost utility ratio £/QALY | |
|---|---|---|
| Paired comparisons | Societal perspective | Ministry of Health perspective |
| Sumatriptan oral tablets versus: | | |
| oral ergotamine/caffeine | £3,000 ($7,500) | £11,760 ($29,400) |
| ASA plus metoclopramide | £3,880 ($9,700) | £18,880 ($47,200) |

£1= $2.5
*Source:* Canadian Co-ordinating Office for Health Technology Assessment (1997)

Cost-effectiveness analysis indicates that the additional costs to the NHS in England associated with increasing triptan use for migraine are potentially considerable. If half of the 3 per cent currently diagnosed with migraine in primary care were switched to oral sumatriptan, this would cost the NHS £114 million for the drug alone. A worse case scenario could be for half of all 12 per cent of predicted migraineux to receive oral sumatriptan at a cost of £456 million. Significant savings to the NHS from the reduction in the use of secondary care services are unlikely.

A stratified approach to therapy is likely to be more cost-effective (Ferrari 1998a). However, applying a stratified care approach to migraine, identifying the 25 per cent of migraine sufferers with significant disability (Sawyer *et al.* 1998) would lead to increased costs of about £57–228 million; this may be offset by greater gains. The cost per aborted attack will depend on the actual efficacy of the triptan, which may vary according to the severity of a person's condition. If, for example, the efficacy was 70 per cent and the drug acquisition cost remained the same, then the additional cost per aborted attack would only be £30.

GPRD data suggest that a significant proportion of migraine sufferers never consult their GPs for their headache. Lipton *et al.* (1998) identified 30–40 per cent under-reporting of migraine in the USA. A large proportion of these patients who had never consulted reported high levels of pain and disability, suggesting that there are opportunities appropriately to increase health care utilisation for migraine. The same is likely to be true for the UK. This emphasises the need to target therapy.

Given the competing pressures for NHS expenditure, it is not clear whether primary care groups (PCGs) will regard migraine therapy as a high enough priority to invest in the relatively expensive triptans. However, there are potential gains in production and the well-being of the individuals receiving the triptans. This raises the question of who should pay? Walley (1998) in a recent editorial in the *BMJ* proposed a reform of the current prescription charge levied in the UK with a move towards a charge based on a drug's effectiveness, a system operated by several other countries. He suggested four lists against which the proportion of co-payment would vary.

Whereas aspirin plus metoclopramide would be considered to be a 'list A' medicine (effective essential drugs), the triptans could be considered to fall within 'list B' as medicines that are no more effective than list A medicines or offer minor benefits at a disproportionate cost. A low co-payment would be recommended related to the cost of the prescription.

## Conclusions

This analysis has identified that controlled trials on resource utilisation and outcomes with the triptans compared to conventional prescription therapy are required. These are essential for accurate assessment of the health economic consequences associated with treatment. A UK-based cost-utility study is required urgently, particularly with the advent of PCGs, the introduction of an integrated health care budget and a more managed care approach.

### Acknowledgements

We would like to thank the Prescription Pricing Authority for their permission to publish the West Midlands PACT data contained in this chapter. Likewise, we are grateful to the Department of Health for the opportunity to present an analysis based on GPRD data.

## *References*

Anon (1996). Drug treatments for migraine. *Bandolier* **33**, 2–4.

Block G, Kramer M, Smith D *et al.* (1998). *Efficacy and safety of rizatriptan vs standard care during long-term treatment.* Merck Research Laboratories Rizatriptan Investigators Meeting, 15.

Canadian Co-ordinating Office for Health Technology Assessment (1997). *An economic analysis of sumatriptan for acute migraine.* CCOHTA publications, Ottawa.

Daly M & Hurst BC (1998). *PC-based health economic model in migraine – case studies.* Presented at the 3rd European Federation of Neurological Societies, 19–25 September 1998.

Drummond MF, O'Brien B, Stoddart GL & Torrance GW (ed.) (1997). *Methods for the economic evaluation of health care programmes* 2 edn. Oxford University Press, Oxford.

European Commission (1998). *Notice to applicants. Medicinal products for human use.* 4.2, 19.

Ferrari M (1998a). The economic burden of migraine to society. *Pharmacoeconomics* **13**(6), 667–76.

Ferrari M (1998b). Migraine: a seminar. *Lancet* **351**, 1043–51.

Frischer M & Chapman S (1998). Issues and directions in prescribing analysis. In *Medicines management* (ed. R Panton & S Chapman). BMJ Books & Pharmaceutical Press, London.

Goadsby P (1998). A triptan too far? *J Neurol Neurosurg Psychiatry* **64**, 143–7.

Gross MLP, Dowson AJ, Deavy L & Duthie T (1996). Impact of oral sumatriptan on work productivity and quality of life in migraineurs. *British Journal of Medical Economics* **10**, 231–46.

Lipton R B (1998). *Oral Presentation of UK Migraine Prevalence Telephone Survey using HIS diagnostic criteria.* European Headache Federation Meeting, Corfu.

Lipton RB, Stewart WF & Simon D (1998). Medical consultation for migraine: results from the American Migraine Study. *Headache* **38**, 87–96.

Mathew NT *et al.* (1997). Naratriptan is effective and well tolerated in the acute treatment of migraine: results of a double-blind, placebo-controlled, crossover study. *Neurology* **49**, 1485–90.

The Multinational Oral Sumatriptan and Cafergot Comparative Study Group (1992). A randomised double blind comparison of sumatriptan and Cafergot in the acute treatment of migraine. *Eur J Neurol* **31**, 314–22.

Mushey GR, Miller D, Clements B *et al.* (1996). Impact of sumatriptan on workplace productivity, nonwork activities, and health-related quality of life among hospital employees with migraine. *Headache* **36**, 137–43.

Myllylä VV, Havanka H, Herrala L, Kangasniemi P, Rautakorpi I, Turkka J *et al.* (1998). Tolfenamic acid rapid release versus sumatriptan in the acute treatment of migraine: comparable effect in a double-blind, randomised, controlled, parallel-group study. *Headache* **38**(3), 201–7.

The Oral Sumatriptan and Aspirin plus Metoclopramide Comparative Study Group (1992). A study to compare oral sumatriptan with oral aspirin and metoclopramide in the acute treatment of migraine. *Eur J Neurol* **32**, 177–84.

Rodríguez LAG & Gutthann SP (1998). Use of the UK General Practice Research Database for pharmacoepidemiology. *Br J Clin Pharmacol* **45**, 419–25.

Sawyer J, Edmeads J, Lipton RB *et al.* (1998). Clinical utility of a new instrument assessing migraine disability: the Migraine Disability Instrument (MIDAS) questionnaire. *Neurology* **50**, A433–4.

Solomon GD & Price KL (1997). Burden of migraine. A review of its socioeconomic impact. *Pharmacoeconomics* **11**(Suppl.1), 1–10.

Stevens A, Colin-Jones D & Gabbay J (1995). Quick and clean: authoritative health technology assessment for local health care contracting. *Health Trends* **27**, 37–42.

Tepper S (1998). *Oral presentation of a US double blind randomised parallel group multiple attack study (ZOMCO), comparing zolmitriptan (2.5 & 5.0mg) with sumatriptan (25 & 50mg) in 1,445 patients treating 6,187 evaluable migraine attacks.* Satellite Symposium EFNS, Seville.

Tepper SJ & Millson DS (1998). The new triptans – 5-HT$_{1B/1D}$ receptor agonists for acute treatment of migraine: a clinical review using NNT. *Eur J Neurol* **59**(Suppl.3), S55.

Tfelt-Hansen P, Henry P, Mulder L J, Schledtewaert R G, Schoenen J & Chazot G (1995). The effectiveness of combined oral lysine acetylsalicylate and metoclopramide compared with oral sumatriptan for migraine. *Lancet* **346**, 923–6.

Tfelt-Hansen P, Teall J, Rodriguez F *et al.* (1998). Earlier onset of action and greater overall efficacy of oral rizatriptan versus oral sumatriptan: a randomised, comparative study in the treatment of migraine. *Headache* (in press).

Visser WH, Terwindt GM, Reines SA Jiang K, Lines CR & Ferrari MD (1996). (Encapsulated) rizatriptan vs. sumatriptan in the acute treatment of migraine. A placebo-controlled, dose ranging study. Dutch/US rizatriptan study. *Arch Neurol* **53**, 1132–7.

Walley T (1998). Prescription charges: change overdue? *BMJ* **317**, 487–8.

Wells N (1998). *Migraine treatment: regaining lost time – new eletriptan study results.* European Headache Federation Meeting, Corfu.

Chapter 9

# Investigation and management of migraine in women

*Anne MacGregor*

## Introduction

All published prevalence studies show migraine to be more common in women than in men. However, migraine is equally common in both sexes before puberty, with increasing female predominance only seen following menarche (Bille 1962). During the reproductive years, prevalence increases in women to peak during the 40s, the time of life when hormonal changes leading to the menopause become apparent (Stewart *et al.* 1992). Epidemiological studies suggest that female-to-male ratio is 3:1, with a lifetime migraine prevalence of 25 per cent for women and 8 per cent for men (Rasmussen *et al.* 1991). There is a decline in migraine in both sexes in later life. Although female sex hormones are the obvious reason to account for this difference between the sexes, the true role of hormones is complex and not fully understood. Hormonal events certainly affect migraine, with improvement and deterioration seen in different women associated with menstruation, use of hormonal contraception, pregnancy, the climacteric, menopause and use of hormone replacement therapy.

## Type of migraine

In addition to gender differences in overall migraine prevalence, there seems to be a difference in hormonal responsiveness between migraine without aura and migraine with aura.

### Migraine without aura

Migraine without aura is more prevalent in women following menarche than migraine with aura (Stewart *et al.* 1991; Rasmussen & Olesen 1992). 'Menstrual' migraine is typically migraine without aura (Somerville 1975a; Lichten *et al.* 1996), as is migraine during the pill-free interval of combined oral contraceptives (MacGregor & Guillebaud 1998). During pregnancy, it is typically migraine without aura that improves (Lance & Anthony 1966; Ratinahirana *et al.* 1990).

### Migraine with aura

In some cases, high oestrogen states are associated with the development of migraine aura in women who have not previously had migraine or had attacks of migraine without aura. This is seen with use of combined oral contraceptives (Bickerstaff

**108** Evidence and treatment

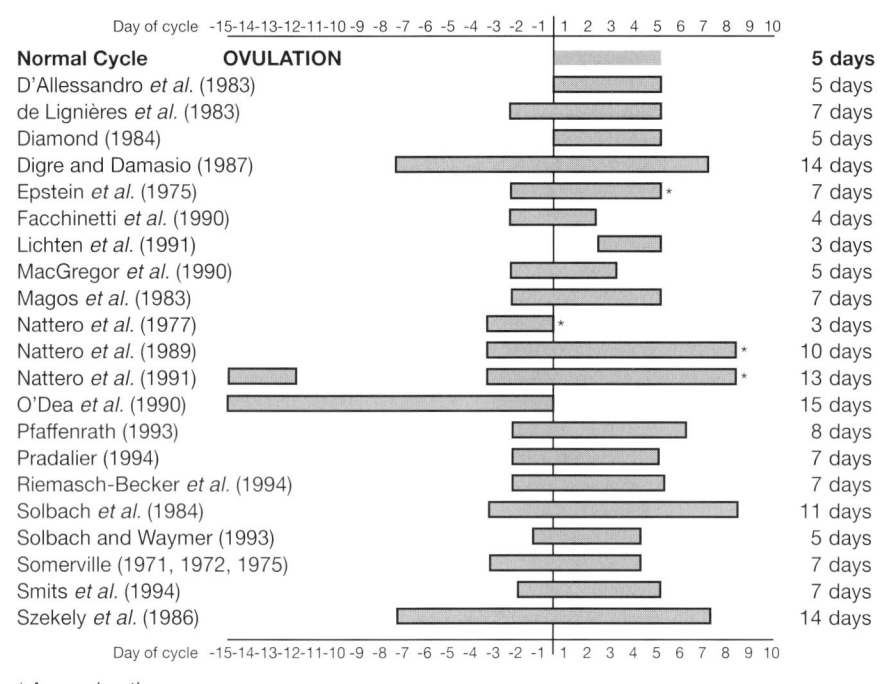

| Study | Day of cycle | Duration |
|---|---|---|
| Normal Cycle (OVULATION) | 1 to 5 | 5 days |
| D'Allessandro et al. (1983) | 1 to 5 | 5 days |
| de Lignières et al. (1983) | -2 to 5 | 7 days |
| Diamond (1984) | 1 to 5 | 5 days |
| Digre and Damasio (1987) | -7 to 7 | 14 days |
| Epstein et al. (1975) | 1 to 7* | 7 days |
| Facchinetti et al. (1990) | -1 to 3 | 4 days |
| Lichten et al. (1991) | 4 to 6 | 3 days |
| MacGregor et al. (1990) | -2 to 3 | 5 days |
| Magos et al. (1983) | -3 to 4 | 7 days |
| Nattero et al. (1977) | -3 to -1* | 3 days |
| Nattero et al. (1989) | -5 to 5* | 10 days |
| Nattero et al. (1991) | -13 to -9, -5 to 3* | 13 days |
| O'Dea et al. (1990) | -14 to -1 | 15 days |
| Pfaffenrath (1993) | -2 to 6 | 8 days |
| Pradalier (1994) | -2 to 5 | 7 days |
| Riemasch-Becker et al. (1994) | -2 to 5 | 7 days |
| Solbach et al. (1984) | -3 to 8 | 11 days |
| Solbach and Waymer (1993) | -1 to 4 | 5 days |
| Somerville (1971, 1972, 1975) | -4 to 3 | 7 days |
| Smits et al. (1994) | -3 to 4 | 7 days |
| Szekely et al. (1986) | -6 to 8 | 14 days |

*Approximation

**Figure 9.1** Variations of definitions of 'menstrual migraine' based on average duration of menstruation of 5 days (*Source*: MacGregor 1996)

1975), hormone replacement therapy (Kaiser & Meienberg 1993) and during pregnancy (Wright & Patel 1986; Chancellor *et al.* 1990). Resolution of aura typically occurs following a return to lower oestrogen states (MacGregor 1999b). Women with migraine with aura are reported to have higher oestrogen levels during the menstrual cycle than those with migraine without aura (Nigel-Leiby *et al.* 1990).

## 'Menstrual' migraine

Many women note that they are more likely to have migraine around the time of their menstrual period. This is particularly the case during the climacteric years, often with little association between migraine and menstruation earlier in the migraine history. There is evidence that migraine in this population, as for migraine in general, is underdiagnosed and undertreated (MacGregor & Barnes 1999). This has important implications since this is also the time of peak employment productivity. Women using combined oral contraceptives may notice migraine occurring during the pill-free interval in association with the withdrawal bleed. This implies that ovulation is not necessary to provoke 'menstrual' attacks.

## Definition

Despite more than 50 per cent of women reporting an association between migraine and menstruation, there is no agreed definition for the term (MacGregor *et al.* 1997). For some it means attacks occurring at the time of ovulation, during menstruation, for a day or two after menstruation, or even premenstrually (MacGregor 1996). Other researchers report migraine more commonly in the week after menstruation (see Figure 9.1).

If research is to uncover mechanisms and treatment for menstrual migraine, there needs to be a standard definition. The Headache Classification Committee of the International Headache Society (1988) has classified most headaches but no definition of menstrual migraine has been agreed:

> *'Migraine without aura may occur almost exclusively at a particular time of the menstrual cycle – so-called menstrual migraine. Generally accepted criteria for this entity are not available. It seems reasonable to demand that 90 per cent of attacks should occur between two days before menses and the last day of menses, but further epidemiological knowledge is needed'.*

In order to provide a more specific definition, women with migraine attending the City of London Migraine Clinic for their first appointment were asked to keep a record of their migraine attacks and menstrual periods for at least three complete menstrual cycles (MacGregor *et al.* 1990). This was a routine part of their treatment programme, in order to remove any potential bias. Records kept by women on the oral contraceptive pill or other hormonal treatments were excluded from the final analysis. The results for all three cycles for every woman were collated and recorded on a graph counting the days forwards and backwards from the first day of menstruation (Figure 9.2). This was done so that the effect of ovulation on migraine, occurring at day –14 (14 days before the onset of menstruation, regardless of cycle length), could be assessed.

From these results we found a marked increase in the number of migraine attacks recorded around the onset of bleeding. These attacks were typically of migraine without aura. Attacks of migraine with aura occurred at other times of the month but no consistent link with menstruation was seen. Further, there was no increase in migraine in association with ovulation. This increase in migraine around day 1 of bleeding and no link with ovulation confirm similar findings from other studies (Waters & O'Connor 1971; Dalton 1973; Johannes *et al.* 1995). Therefore, we proposed the following definition for 'menstrual' migraine: 'Attacks of migraine which occur regularly on day 1 of menstruation ±2 days and at no other time'. According to these criteria, 7 per cent of the women in the study had 'menstrual' migraine. However, even when these patients were excluded from the overall data, the number of attacks

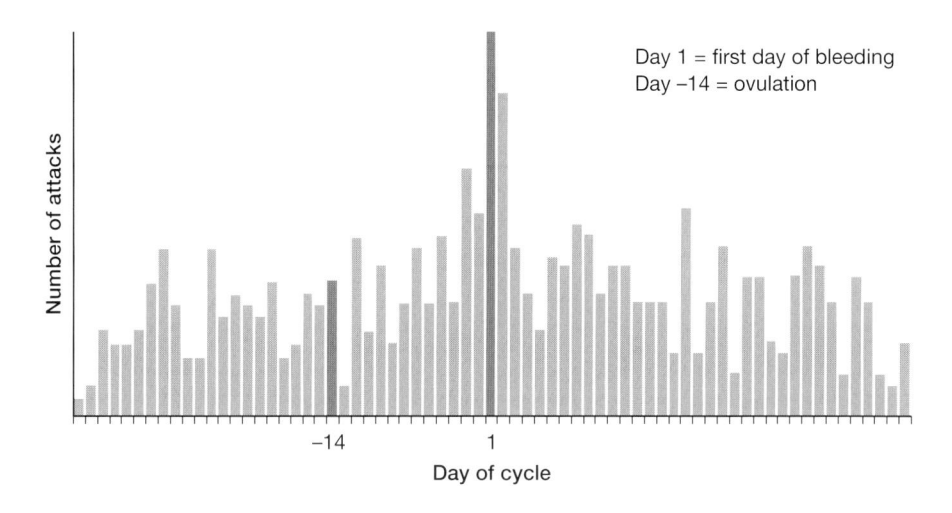

**Figure 9.2** Total number of attacks recorded over 3 complete menstrual cycles by 55 women (*Source*: MacGregor *et al.* 1990)

of migraine occurring around day 1 of menstruation was still higher than at any other time of the cycle. This means that, for many women, menstruation acts as an additional migraine trigger, increasing the overall susceptibility to attacks perimenstrually. Despite this, the definition for 'menstrual' migraine proposes exclusive attacks in order to help identify mechanisms by including only those women with a probable hormonal trigger, excluding women who have additional non-hormonal triggers. This is also important for effective management since only those women with exclusively hormonal triggers are likely to respond to hormonal treatment.

## Mechanisms

What possible mechanism(s) could account for this effect of menstruation on migraine? Numerous mechanisms have been proposed for 'menstrual' migraine, including reduced levels of magnesium (Facchinetti *et al.* 1991), platelet dysfunction (Benedetto *et al.* 1987), and central serotonin dysmodulation (Silberstein & Merriam 1993).

But the most likely cause is some abnormality of hormonal function. Oestrogen and progesterone are the main hormones which have been studied in relation to migraine but studies comparing levels of these hormones in women with 'menstrual' migraine versus controls have not found any convincing differences. Research has therefore focused on the naturally declining level of these hormones which occurs during the luteal phase of the menstrual cycle, coinciding with the onset of 'menstrual' migraine.

## Progesterone withdrawal?

Progesterone has long been considered as a treatment for headache associated with menstruation (Gray 1941; Singh & Singh 1947). However, Somerville treated six women who generally had attacks of migraine during the late luteal phase with progesterone (Somerville 1972). Menstruation was delayed in four of the women but, in spite of this, five experienced migraine at their customary time, unrelated to plasma progesterone levels.

## Oestrogen withdrawal?

The most convincing mechanism to date is that of oestrogen withdrawal, as proposed by Somerville. Somerville treated 14 women, each of whom had a predictable attack of migraine every month always confined to the premenstrual or menstrual phases. Each subject had had an attack for at least six successive cycles immediately prior to the study. A review of the manuscripts shows that all the subjects had attacks occurring on or between days −3 to +4 of the menstrual cycle. On the basis of his observations, Somerville suggested that migraine could be triggered by the sudden withdrawal of oestrogens following several days' exposure to high oestrogen levels.

If this mechanism is correct, stabilising fluctuations by maintaining high, stable levels of oestrogen should prevent migraine. In favour of this, Somerville showed that migraine could be postponed by maintaining high plasma oestradiol levels with an intramuscular injection of long-acting oestradiol valerate in oil; migraine subsequently occurred when the plasma oestradiol fell. The administration of a short-acting oestrogen did not produce the same result, confirming his suggestion that prolonged oestrogen exposure is necessary for withdrawal to trigger migraine. Somerville further attempted to control oestrogen fluctuations with oral oestrogens and oestrogen implants, but both these methods failed to provide stable plasma levels of oestradiol and so, not surprisingly, did not produce an improvement in migraine.

Several other studies support Somerville's oestrogen-withdrawal theory. Lichten *et al.* (1996) studied postmenopausal women challenged with oestrogen confirming that, in some of these women, a drop in serum oestrogen could precipitate migraine and that a period of oestrogen priming was a necessary prerequisite. Dennerstein *et al.* (1978) reported increased frequency of headache when an oestrogen preparation was followed by a non-oestrogen preparation in their double-blind placebo-controlled cross-over study of hysterectomised women with bilateral oophorectomies treated with ethinyloestradiol ± progestogen. Whitty *et al.* (1966) noted migraine during the pill-free week of combined oral contraceptives. Migraine has also been shown to occur in the now-redundant regimen of cyclical oestrogen replacement therapy (Kudrow 1975).

Epstein *et al.* (1975) suggested that variation in hormonal activity might be a potentially relevant factor in *all* women with migraine; their biochemical studies showed similar results for menstrual migraine and non-menstrual migraine patients.

They concluded that factors additional to the hormonal environment must be responsible for the difference between the subgroups of women with migraine. Certainly, the regulation of the menstrual cycle is complex with ovarian steroids playing a limited role in the overall control. Furthermore, other events associated with menstruation have been shown to be associated with migraine, in particular, prostaglandin release.

### Prostaglandin release

Entry of prostaglandins into the systemic circulation can trigger throbbing headache, nausea and vomiting (Carlson *et al.* 1968). With regard to the menstrual cycle, there is a three-fold increase in prostaglandin levels in the uterine endometrium from the follicular to the luteal phase, with a further increase during menstruation (Speroff *et al.* 1994). Maximal entry of prostaglandins and prostaglandin metabolites into the systemic circulation occurs during the first 48 hours of menstruation. This mechanism is most likely to be relevant to attacks occurring after the onset of menstruation, particularly in association with menorrhagia and/or dysmenorrhoea (Benedetto 1989).

### Investigations

Since no hormonal or biochemical abnormalities have been identified in 'menstrual' migraine, there is no place for specific investigations other than those which may be required in usual clinical practice when indicated to exclude secondary headache resulting from underlying pathology.

## Management of suspected 'menstrual' migraine

### First consultation

Once the diagnosis of migraine has been established, management strategies should include acute therapies, advice on non-hormonal trigger factors, and the provision of diary cards.

### Attack therapy

Effective attack therapy may be all that is required if attacks are only occurring once a month. Standard acute treatments are effective (Solbach & Waymer 1993; Facchinetti *et al.* 1995; Dalessio *et al.* 1996; Loder 1998; MacGregor 1998; Silberstein *et al.* 1998). However, there is some evidence that in women with menstrually related migraine, attacks linked to menstruation are less responsive to treatment compared to migraine at other times of the cycle (Gross *et al.* 1995). Also, recurrence of symptoms is more likely in 'menstrual' attacks. One possible reason for this is the longer duration of the 'menstrual' trigger. In these cases, ergotamine with its longer duration of action and lower recurrence may be the drug of choice (British Association for the Study of Headache 1999).

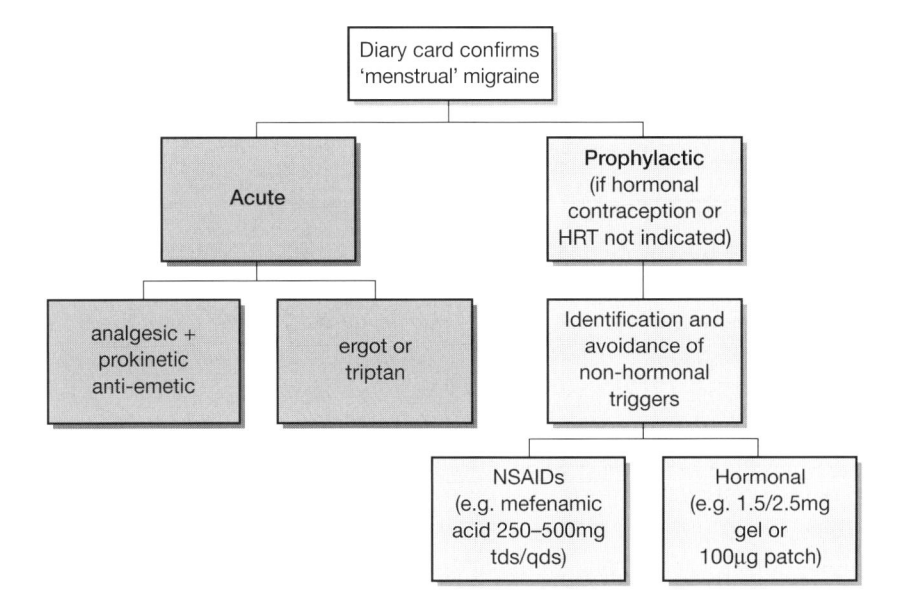

**Figure 9.3** Management of menstrual migraine in women with regular menses who do not require hormonal contraception

### Identification of non-hormonal triggers

Assuming the concept of multiple factors acting in combination to trigger migraine, hormonal factors combine with non-hormonal triggers to increase the overall susceptibility to attacks at the time of menstruation (Amery & Vandenbergh 1987). Therefore, every effort should be made to identify and eliminate non-hormonal triggers. In some cases, this may reduce the frequency and severity of all attacks. In others, non-hormonal attacks are eliminated, while 'menstrual' attacks persist.

### Diary cards

The most important aspect of management is to establish a true link between migraine and menstruation. Simple diary cards, on which attacks of migraine and menstruation are recorded for a minimum of three menstrual cycles, can be used to confirm or refute the association.

## Subsequent consultation

By the time the diary cards are reviewed at follow-up, a percentage of patients will have their attacks under control, with no need for further intervention. Another group will have attacks throughout the cycle which are not obviously related to menstruation. These women may benefit from standard prophylactic therapy, if considered necessary.

Only a small percentage of women will have 'menstrual' migraine requiring specific prophylaxis. Depending on each woman's wishes, the regularity of the menstrual cycle, timing of attacks in relation to bleeding, presence of dysmenorrhoea or menorrhagia, presence of menopausal symptoms, or need for contraception, several options can be tried, both non-hormonal and hormonal.

## Specific prophylaxis for 'menstrual' migraine

None of the drugs and hormones recommended is licensed for management of menstrual migraine and there is little evidence for their efficacy. Therefore, an empirical approach is necessary, with each regimen used for three cycles before being deemed ineffective.

### Non-steroidal anti-inflammatory drugs (NSAIDs)

NSAIDs are effective prostaglandin inhibitors. They should be tried as first-line agents for migraine attacks that start on the first-to-third day of bleeding, particularly in the presence of dysmenorrhoea and/or menorrhagia. Side-effects include gastrointestinal disturbance. Contraindications include peptic ulcer and aspirin-induced allergy. Interactions include anticoagulants and antihypertensive agents.

**Mefenamic acid** is probably the drug of choice as it is particularly helpful in reducing associated menorrhagia and/or dysmenorrhoea; however, no clinical trials have been undertaken in menstrual migraine (Owens 1984). The dose is 500 mg 3–4 times daily. This should be started either 2–3 days before the expected onset of menstruation, or started on the first day of bleeding and this should be taken for 2–3 days when bleeding is heavy, but can be used for the duration of menstrual bleeding.

Some studies have suggested **naproxen** 550 mg once or twice daily from 7 days before menstruation for a total of 14 days, although other studies refute the drug's efficacy (Sances *et al.* 1990; Nattero *et al.* 1991). Alternatively, **fenoprofen** 600 mg has been tried, taken twice daily from 3 days before the onset of menstruation until the last day of bleeding (Diamond 1984).

### Triptans

Although one open study of prophylactic oral sumatriptan given perimenstrually showed good results preventing 'menstrual' attacks, prophylactic use of triptans is not recommended until results of double-blind placebo-controlled trials are available (Newman *et al.* 1998).

### Oestrogen supplements

**Percutaneous oestrogen supplements.** Trials of treatment for 'menstrual' migraine using oestrogen supplementation with percutaneous gel to prevent fluctuations have shown some efficacy. De Lignières *et al.* (1986) studied 18 women with strictly defined 'menstrual' migraine who completed a double-blind placebo-controlled cross-over trial using 1.5 mg oestradiol gel (which allows a mean oestradiol plasma level of 80 pg/ml to be reached) or placebo daily for 7 days during 3 consecutive cycles. Treatment was started 48 hours before the earliest expected onset of migraine. Only 8 menstrual attacks occurred during the 26 oestrogen-treated cycles (30.8 per cent) compared to 26 attacks during the 27 placebo cycles (96.3 per cent). Further, attacks during oestrogen treatment were considerably milder and shorter than those during placebo.

Eighteen women also completed a similar trial by Dennerstein *et al.* (1988): 1.5 mg oestradiol gel or placebo was used daily for 7 days, beginning at least 2 days prior to the expected migraine, for 4 cycles. The difference between oestradiol gel and placebo was highly significant and less medication was used during active treatment. However, the results were not as impressive as the study by De Lignières *et al.* (1986). Dennerstein *et al.* comment that the reason for this may be that women in their group also experienced migraine at other times of the cycle and therefore their migraine was only partially hormone-dependent.

**Transdermal oestrogen supplements.** Trials with oestrogen patches have not been as successful in preventing migraine. Pfaffenrath (1993) studied 41 patients completing a trial of 50 μg oestradiol patches versus placebo used daily from 2 days prior to the suspected onset of migraine, during a 4-month treatment phase. No significant differences were seen between the two treatments, although oestradiol was slightly better in all parameters. Smits *et al.* (1994) also used 50 μg patches versus placebo over 3 cycles in 20 women. They also found no difference between oestradiol and placebo. Pradalier *et al.* (1994) studied 2 groups of 12 women using either 25 μg or 100 μg patches on day –4 and day 0 (2 patches per cycle) over 2 cycles and compared the results to a pre-treatment cycle. They found that the 100 μg patches gave a better clinical result than the 25 μg ones, raising the question of a critical level. The suggestion is that the 25 μg and 50 μg patches are not effective in preventing 'menstrual' migraine, as they produce suboptimal doses of supplemental oestrogen with oestradiol serum levels of 25 pg/ml and 40 pg/ml respectively; the 100 μg patch effectively produces higher plasma oestradiol levels of 75 pg/ml, similar to serum levels attained using the 1.5 mg percutaneous oestradiol used by de Lignières *et al.* and Dennerstein *et al.*

**Oestrogen supplements in practice.** Perimenstrual oestrogen supplements for migraine prophylaxis can only be used when menstruation is regular and predictable. Although these regimens use treatments normally given for hormone replacement therapy, it is important to note that for 'menstrual' migraine, hormones are given as supplements. Provided the woman is ovulating regularly, no additional progestogens are necessary. This is because she will be producing adequate amounts of her own natural progesterone to counter the effects of unopposed oestrogen, which could otherwise lead to endometrial proliferation and hyperplasia. Ovulation can be confirmed, if necessary, with blood levels of progesterone taken 7 days before expected menstruation, i.e. day 21 of a 28-day cycle. The level should be greater than 30 mmol/l (Hardiman & Ginsburg 1996). Side-effects due to excess oestrogen include breast tenderness, fluid retention, nausea and leg cramps.

**Transdermal oestrogen 100 µg** or **oestradiol gel 1.5 mg in 2.5 g gel** can be used from approximately 2–3 days before expected menstruation for about 5–7 days. If this is effective but side-effects are a problem, lower doses can subsequently be tried.

Oestrogen supplements should not be used by women who are at risk of pregnancy, have undiagnosed vaginal bleeding, or oestrogen-dependent tumours.

## Continuous hormonal strategies

If cycles are irregular, or the above strategies are ineffective despite a convincing hormonal link, the following methods can be considered. Several of these regimens are contraceptive.

**Combined oral contraception** (COC) inhibits ovulation, producing fairly stable oestrogen levels when taken, and can improve migraine in some women. Standard COC prescribing recommendations should be followed. The UK recommendations follow the WHO guidelines, contraindicating COC in women with migraine with aura (World Health Organization 1996; MacGregor & Guillebaud 1998). Migraine without aura occurring a couple of days into the pill-free interval can be controlled by use of three consecutive packets, thus reducing the number of breaks from 13 to 5 per year (MacGregor & Guillebaud 1998). Alternatively, oestrogen supplements can be used, as for 'menstrual' migraine (unpublished data).

**Levonorgestrel-releasing (Mirena) intrauterine system** (IUS) is licensed for contraception but is also highly effective at reducing menstrual bleeding and associated pain. It can be considered for migraine related to dysmenorrhoea and/or menorrhagia (Rybo 1998). It is not effective for women who are sensitive to oestrogen withdrawal as a migraine trigger, as the majority of women still ovulate with the system *in situ*. Systemic effects are usually minor but erratic bleeding and spotting are common in the early months of use. Most women are amenorrhoeic within one year.

**Injectable depot progestogens** inhibit ovulation, similar to the mode of action of COC. Although irregular, bleeding can occur in early months of treatment; this method has the advantage that in most cases menstruation ceases. By eventually inhibiting the normal menstrual cycle, hormonal triggers are removed. This should confer efficacy in 'menstrual' migraine, although no clinical trial data are available.

**Oestradiol implants** are the most effective method of obtaining high stable oestrogen levels. Magos *et al.* (1983) showed that implant doses large enough to suppress ovulation and produce constant plasma oestrogen levels achieved a 96 per cent response rate in 24 patients studied. However, in unhysterectomised women, progestogen opposition is necessary to protect the endometrium.

**Oral progestogen-only contraception** has little place in the management of 'menstrual' migraine. It has no effect on potential mechanisms for 'menstrual' migraine, does not inhibit ovulation and is associated with a disrupted menstrual cycle (Chumnijaraki et al. 1984).

**Gonadotrophin-releasing hormones** have been tried but side-effects of oestrogen deficiency (e.g. hot flushes) restrict their use. They are also associated with a marked reduction in bone density and should not be used for longer than six months without regular monitoring and bone densitometry. 'Add back' continuous combined oestrogen and progestogen can be given to counter these difficulties (Holdaway et al. 1991; Murray & Muse 1997). Given these limitations, in addition to increased cost, such treatment is best instigated in specialist departments.

**Hysterectomy** has no place in the management of migraine alone. Studies show that migraine is more likely to deteriorate after surgical menopause with bilateral oophorectomy (Dalton 1956; Neri et al. 1993). However, if other medical problems require surgical menopause, the effects on migraine are probably lessened by subsequent oestrogen replacement therapy, as for natural menopause.

## Hormone replacement therapy and migraine

If cycles are of irregular nature and associated with menopausal symptoms, hormone replacement therapy (HRT) should be considered. It is a commonly held belief that HRT will aggravate migraine. This is certainly true if HRT is prescribed without consideration of the potential hormonal triggering mechanisms of migraine.

### Oestrogen

Studies suggest that non-oral routes of delivery of oestrogen are more likely to improve migraine than oral ones (Erkkola et al. 1991; Evans et al. 1995; MacGregor 1999a). Oral oestrogens are associated with wide day-to-day variations in serum concentrations, which could play a part in triggering migraine, particularly if coupled with a background of fluctuating endogenous oestrogens in perimenopausal women. Conversely, non-oral routes, such as transdermal or percutaneous routes, are associated with more stable oestrogen levels at physiologic doses. Tailoring treatment is particularly difficult for perimenopausal women as too high a dose, coupled with surges of endogenous oestrogen, can trigger migraine aura as well as causing symptoms of oestrogen excess, including nausea, fluid retention, breast tenderness and leg cramps.

### Progestogens

Additional progestogen is necessary to prevent endometrial cancer in unhysterectomised women using oestrogen replacement. However, side-effects are common, including perimenstrual symptoms, headaches and migraine (Magos et al. 1986; Vestergaard et al. 1997). Clinically, this appears to be more of a problem with cyclical progestogens than with continuous combined regimens, although there are no studies to confirm this. The latter is only indicated for postmenopausal women. Changing the type of progestogen can resolve the problem, as side-effects are fewer with progesterone derivatives such as medroxyprogesterone acetate and dydrogesterone than with testosterone derivatives such as norethisterone (Panay & Studd 1998). Changing route from oral to transdermal progestogen may also be effective. The course of cyclical progestogens could be reduced to only 7–10 days per month, although this increases the risk of endometrial hyperplasia (Lane *et al.* 1988). Alternatively, if natural periods are infrequent, progestogens could be limited to three-monthly cycles. Natural progesterone is available as suppositories and, in some countries, as micronised tablets. However, sedation is a common side-effect when progesterone is absorbed systemically. Progesterone vaginal gel is useful in these situations. The levonorgestrel-releasing intrauterine system (Mirena) can provide the progestogen component with minimal systemic effects, although it is not yet licensed for this indication (Suhonen 1998). Occasionally, progestogenic side-effects are sufficient for a woman to choose to discontinue progestogens. In these cases, specialist care is appropriate because of the risk of endometrial hyperplasia and cancer.

## Non-hormonal prophylaxis

Clonidine (50–75 μg b.d.) is licensed for menopausal hot flushes and migraine prophylaxis and may be useful for women unwilling, or unable, to take HRT. However, trial data to support its efficacy as a migraine prophylactic are limited (Anon 1990). Side-effects include sedation, dry mouth, dizziness and insomnia. As it is also anti-hypertensive, it should not be taken concomitantly with other anti-hypertensive agents.

## Conclusions

Although hormonal events affect migraine, there is rarely a need for hormonal intervention, as effective acute treatment may suffice. For frequent migraine, standard prophylactic regimens are appropriate. The need for specific hormonal strategies should be evidenced from diary cards. In these cases, several options are available depending on factors such as associated menstrual symptoms, timing of attacks, need for contraception and presence or absence of menopausal symptoms.

### *References*

Amery WK & Vandenbergh V (1987). What can precipitating factors teach us about the pathogenesis of migraine? *Headache* **27**, 146–50.

Anonymous (1990). Clonidine in migraine prophylaxis – now obsolete. *Drugs and Therapeutics Bulletin* **28**, 79–80.

Benedetto C (1989). Eicosanoids in primary dysmenorrhea, endometriosis and menstrual migraine. *Gynecol Endocrinol* **3**, 71–94.

Benedetto C, Massobrio M, Zonca M, Melzi E, Nattero G, Allais G & Torre E (1987). Menstrual migraine: a possible pathogenic implication of platelet function. *Gynaecol Endocrinol* **1**, 345–53.

Bickerstaff ER (1975). *Neurological complications of oral contraceptives.* Oxford University Press, Oxford.

Bille B (1962). Migraine in school-children. *Acta Paed Scand* **51** (Suppl.136), 1–151.

British Association for the Study of Headache (1999). *Guidelines for all doctors in the diagnosis and management of migraine.* British Association for the Study of Headache, London.

Carlson LA, Ekelund L-G & Orö L (1968). Clinical and metabolic effects of different doses of prostaglandin E1 in man. *Acta Med Scand* **183**, 423–30.

Chancellor AM, Wroe SJ & Cull RE (1990). Migraine occurring for the first time in pregnancy. *Headache* **30**, 224–7.

Chumnijaraki T, Sunyavivat S, Onthuam Y & Udomprasetgurl V (1984). Study on the factors associated with contraception discontinuation in Bangkok. *Contraception* **29**, 241–8.

Dalessio DJ, Brown DL, Solbach P et al. (1996). Oral 311C90 is effective in the treatment of menstrual migraine. *Cephalalgia* **16**, 400–1.

Dalton K (1956). Discussion on the aftermath of hysterectomy and oophorectomy. *Proc Roy Soc Med* **50**, 415–8.

Dalton K (1973). Progesterone suppositories and pessaries in the treatment of menstrual migraine. *Headache* **13**, 151–9.

De Lignières C, Vincens M, Mauvais-Jarvis P et al. (1986). Prevention of menstrual migraine by percutaneous oestradiol. *BMJ* **293**, 1450.

Dennerstein L, Laby B, Burrows GD & Hyman GJ (1978). Headache and sex hormone therapy. *Headache* **18**, 146–53.

Dennerstein L, Morse C, Burrows G et al. (1988). Menstrual migraine: a double-blind trial of percutaneous estradiol. *Gynaecol Endocrinol* **2**, 113–20.

Diamond S (1984). Menstrual migraine and non-steroidal anti-inflammatory agents. *Headache* **24**, 52.

Epstein MT, Hockaday JM & Hockaday TDR (1975). Migraine and reproductive hormones throughout the menstrual cycle. *Lancet* **1**, 543–8.

Erkkola R, Holma P, Jarvi T et al. (1991). Transdermal oestrogen replacement in a Finnish population. *Maturitas* **13**, 275–81.

Evans MP, Fleming KC & Evans JM (1995). Hormone replacement therapy: management of common problems. *Mayo Clin Proc* **70**, 800–5.

Facchinetti F, Sances G, Borella P, Genazzani AR & Nappi G (1991). Magnesium prophylaxis of menstrual migraine: effects on intracellular magnesium. *Headache* **31**, 298–301.

Facchinetti F, Bonellie G, Kangasniemi P et al. (1995). The efficacy and safety of subcutaneous sumatriptan in the acute treatment of menstrual migraine. *Obstet Gynecol* **86**, 911–16.

Gray LA (1941). The use of progesterone in nervous tension states. *Southern Med J* **34**, 1004–5.

Gross M, Barrie M, Bates D et al. (1995). The efficacy of sumatriptan in menstrual migraine. *Eur J Neurol* **2**, 144–5.

Hardiman P & Ginsburg J (1996). Induction of ovulation. In *Drug therapy in reproductive endocrinology* (ed. J Ginsburg). Arnold, London.

Headache Classification Committee of the International Headache Society (1988). Classification and diagnostic criteria for headache disorders, cranial neuralgias and facial pain. *Cephalalgia* **8** (Suppl.7), 1–96.

Holdaway IM, Parr CE & France J (1991). Treatment of a patient with severe menstrual migraine using the depot LHRH analogue Zoladex. *Aust NZ J Obstet Gynaecol* **31**, 164–5.

Johannes CB, Linet MA, Stewart WF *et al.* (1995). Relationship of headache to phase of the menstrual cycle among young women: a daily diary study. *Neurology* **45**, 1076–82.

Kaiser HJ & Meienberg O (1993). Deterioration of onset of migraine under oestrogen replacement therapy in the menopause. *J Neurol* **240**, 195–7.

Kudrow L (1975). The relationship of headache frequency to hormone use in migraine. *Headache* **15**, 36–49.

Lance JW & Anthony M (1966). Some clinical aspects of migraine. *Arch Neurol* **15**, 356–61.

Lane G, King R & Whitehead MI (1988). The effects of oestrogens and progestogens on endometrial biochemistry. In *The menopause* (ed. JWW Studd & MI Whitehead), pp.213–26. Blackwell Scientific, Oxford.

Lichten E, Lichten J, Whitty A & Pieper D (1996). The confirmation of a biochemical marker for women's hormonal migraine: the depo-oestradiol challenge test. *Headache* **36**, 367–71.

Loder E (1998). Clinical efficacy of 2.5 mg and 5 mg zolmitriptan ('Zomig') in migraine associated with menses or in patients using non-progesterone oral contraceptives. *Neurology* **50** (Suppl.4), 341.

MacGregor EA (1996). 'Menstrual' migraine: towards a definition. *Cephalalgia* **16**, 11–21.

MacGregor EA (1998). Evaluating migraine during menstruation and the potential efficacy of oral eletriptan. *Eur J Neurol* **5** (Suppl.3), S56–7.

MacGregor EA (1999a). Effects of oral and transdermal estrogen replacement on migraine. *Cephalalgia* **19**, 124–5.

MacGregor EA (1999b). Estrogen replacement and migraine aura. *Headache* (in press).

MacGregor EA & Barnes DS (1999). Migraine in a specialist menopause clinic. *Climacteric* (in press).

MacGregor EA & Guillebaud J (1998). Recommendations for clinical practice. Combined oral contraceptives, migraine and ischaemic stroke. *J Fam Planning* **24**, 53–60.

MacGregor EA, Chia HMY, Vohrah C & Wilkinson M (1990). Migraine and menstruation: a pilot study. *Cephalalgia* **10**, 305–10.

MacGregor EA, Igarashi H & Wilkinson M (1997). Headaches and hormones: subjective versus objective assessment. *Headache Quarterly* **8**, 126–36.

Magos AL, Zilkha KJ & Studd JWW (1983). Treatment of menstrual migraine by oestradiol implants. *J Neurol Neurosurg Psychiat* **46**, 1044–6.

Magos AL, Brewster E, Singh R *et al.* (1986). The effects of norethisterone in postmenopausal women on oestrogen replacement therapy: a model for the premenstrual syndrome. *Br J Obstet Gynaecol* **93**, 1290–6.

Murray SC & Muse KN (1997). Effective treatment of severe menstrual migraine headaches with gonadotrophon-releasing hormone agonist and 'add-back' therapy. *Fertil Steril* **67**, 390–3.

Nattero G, Allais G, De Lorenzo C *et al.* (1991). Biological and clinical effects of naproxen sodium in patients with menstrual migraine. *Cephalalgia* **11** (Suppl.11), 201–2.

Neri I, Granella F, Nappi R *et al.* (1993). Characteristics of headache at menopause: a clinico-epidemiologic study. *Maturitas* **17**, 31–7.

Newman LC, Lipton RB, Lay CL & Solomon S (1998). A pilot study of oral sumatriptan as intermittent prophylaxis of menstruation-related migraine. *Neurology* **51**, 307–9.

Nigel-Leiby S, Welch KMA, Grunfeld S & D'Andrea G (1990). Ovarian steroid levels in migraine with and without aura. *Cephalalgia* **10**, 147–52.

Owens PR (1984). Prostaglandin synthetase inhibitors in the treatment of primary dysmenorrhoea: outcome trials reviewed. *Am J Obstet Gynecol* **148**, 96.

Panay N & Studd J (1998). Progestogen side-effects. *The Diplomate* **5**, 37–45.

Pfaffenrath V (1993). Efficacy and safety of percutaneous estradiol vs. placebo in menstrual migraine. *Cephalalgia* **13** (Suppl.13), 244.

Pradalier A, Vincent D, Beaulieu PH *et al.* (1994). Correlation between oestradiol plasma level and therapeutic effect on menstrual migraine. In *New advances in headache research* (ed. FC Rose). Smith-Gordon, London.

Rasmussen BK & Olesen J (1992). Migraine with aura and migraine without aura: an epidemiological study. *Cephalalgia* **12**, 221–8.

Rasmussen BK, Jensen R, Schroll M & Olesen J (1991). Epidemiology of headache in a general population: a prevalence study. *J Clin Epidemiol* **44**, 1147–57.

Ratinahirana H, Darbois Y & Bousser MG (1990). Migraine and pregnancy: a prospective study in 703 women after delivery. *Neurology* **40** (Suppl.1), 437.

Rybo G (1998). Treatment of menorrhagia using intrauterine administration of levonergestrel. *Gynaecology Forum* **3**, 20–2.

Sances G, Martignoni E, Fioroni L *et al.* (1990). Naproxen sodium in menstrual migraine prophylaxis: a double-blind placebo-controlled study. *Headache* **30**, 705–9.

Silberstein SD & Merriam GR (1993). Sex hormones and headache. *J Pain Symptom Manage* **8**, 98–114.

Silberstein SD, Armellino JJ, Hoffman HD *et al.* (1998). Successful treatment of menstruation-associated migraine with a nonprescription combination of acetaminophen, aspirin and caffeine: results from three randomised, placebo-controlled studies. *Neurology* **50**, A376.

Singh I & Singh I (1947). Progesterone in the treatment of migraine. *Lancet* **i**, 745–7.

Smits MG, van der Meer YG, Pfeil JPJM *et al.* (1994). Perimenstrual migraine: effect of Estraderm TTS and the value of contingent negative variation and exteroceptive temporalis muscle suppression test. *Headache* **34**, 103–6.

Solbach MP & Waymer RS (1993). Treatment of menstruation-associated migraine headache with subcuntaneous sumatriptan. *Obstet Gynecol* **82**, 769–72.

Somerville BW (1971). The role of progesterone in menstrual migraine. *Neurology* **21**, 853–9.

Somerville BW (1972). The role of estradiol withdrawal in the etiology of menstrual migraine. *Neurology* **22**, 355–65.

Somerville BW (1975a). Estrogen-withdrawal migraine. *Neurology* **25**, 239–50.

Somerville BW (1975b). Estrogen-withdrawal migraine. 1. Duration of exposure required and attempted prophylaxis by premenstrual estrogen administration. *Neurology* **25**, 239–44.

Somerville BW (1975c). Estrogen-withdrawal migraine. 2. Attempted prophylaxis by continuous estradiol administration. *Neurology* **25**, 245–50.

Speroff L, Glass RH & Kase NG (1994). *Clinical gynecologic endocrinology and infertility*. Williams and Wilkins, Baltimore.

Stewart WF, Linet MA, Celentano DD *et al.* (1991). Age- and sex-specific incidence rates of migraine with and without visual aura. *Am J Epidemiol* **134**, 1111–20.

Stewart WF, Lipton RB, Celentano DD *et al.* (1992). Prevalence of migraine headache in the United States. Relation to age, income, race, and other sociodemographic factors. *JAMA* **267**, 64–9.

Suhonen S (1998). Continuous combined hormone replacement therapy using the levonergestrel-releasing intrauterine system in peri- and postmenopausal women. *Gynaecology Forum* **3**, 29–31.

Vestergaard P, Pernille Hermann A, Gram J *et al.* (1997). Improving compliance with hormonal replacement therapy in primary osteoporosis prevention. *Maturitas* **28**, 137–45.

Waters WE & O'Connor PJ (1971). Epidemiology of headache and migraine in women. *J Neurol Neurosurg Psychiat* **34**, 148–53.

Whitty CWM, Hockaday JM & Whitty MM (1966). The effect of oral contraceptives on migraine. *Lancet* **1**, 856–9.
World Health Organization (1996). *Improving access to quality care in family planning. Medical eligibility criteria for initiating and continuing use of contraceptive methods.* WHO, Geneva.
Wright GDS & Patel MK (1986). Focal migraine and pregnancy. *BMJ* **293**, 1557–8.

## *Further Reading*

MacGregor A (1999). *Managing migraine in primary care.* Blackwell Science, Oxford.
MacGregor A (1999). *Migraine in women.* Martin Dunitz, London.

Chapter 10

# Investigation and management of migraine in childhood

*John Wilson*

## Introduction

Headache is common in childhood. Asked specifically, 8 per cent of children of 3 years (Zuckerman *et al.* 1987) and 19.5 per cent of children of 5 years (Sillanpää *et al.* 1991) will say that they get headaches. Bille (1962) recorded a prevalence of 59 per cent in Swedish school-children. It is probable that the shrill cry and irritability on handling of infants who have had a traumatic delivery indicate that they too can suffer from headache.

Headache is a frequent accompaniment of acute febrile illness and may have ominous significance especially when, associated with fever, vomiting and neck stiffness, it can be a marker for meningitis and meningo-encephalitis. (But neck stiffness may not be obvious in infants.)

This chapter will concentrate on headache as a recurrent symptom with special reference to migraine in childhood.

## Migraine in childhood

Contrary to popular belief, migraine is comparatively frequent in children. Using the International Headache Society criteria for diagnosis, 1.4 per cent of Swedish 7-year-olds and 5.3 per cent of 15-year-olds were considered to suffer from migraine (Bille 1962). In a more recent UK study, 10.6 per cent of school-children (5–15 years) were diagnosed as migraine sufferers (Abu-Arafeh & Russell 1994). The difference in prevalence suggested by these figures could reflect differences in ascertainment but may also indicate an increased incidence. This is suggested by a longitudinal study showing that in Finland the prevalence of migraine in 7-year-old children increased from 1.9 per cent to 5.7 per cent between 1974 and 1992 (Sillanpää & Anttila 1996).

In acknowledging similarities to migraine in adults, as defined by criteria for diagnosis which are adopted in epidemiological surveys, there are some important differences, mainly in respect of the duration of headaches. In children complaint of headache in what appear to be otherwise typical migraine attacks is often much briefer than in adults, although at the other extreme, as in adults, something akin to *status migrainosus* can also occur. By the criteria of the IHS definition, many children would be excluded, but adoption of these criteria without modification is unnecessarily Procrustean in its approach, since affected children have all of the other accompanying symptoms of migraine which are identified in adults (Winner *et al.* 1995). Although it may be lateralised, migraine headache in children is commonly ill defined and frontal; however, lack of lateralisation when all other features are considered is not, in my opinion, justification for excluding the diagnosis.

Of more striking significance are several paramigrainous syndromes which are much more frequent in children than in adults. They include: abdominal migraine; cyclical vomiting; periodic syndrome; benign paroxysmal vertigo; benign paroxysmal torticollis; benign limb pains; recurrent epistaxis; and travel sickness.

## Abdominal migraine

In this syndrome, epigastric pain – often of a persistent and gnawing quality – is more prominent than headache, although as children age, headaches develop, and some children will describe 'headache in my tummy' (Abu-Arafeh & Russell 1995). Often accompanied by pallor, nausea or vomiting, anorexia and malaise, symptoms are the cause of much parental anxiety as in other paramigrainous syndromes.

## Cyclical vomiting

As the name suggests, recurrent nausea and vomiting are predominant symptoms in this condition, which is probably a variant of abdominal migraine (Symon & Russell 1995). In the days before fluid and electrolyte balance were understood and well managed, some children died. The disorder appears to be less frequent nowadays in hospital practice, possibly reflecting the ready availability of effective anti-emetic drugs.

Before diagnosing cyclical vomiting as a paramigrainous syndrome, metabolic disorders such as organic acidaemia (e.g. maple syrup urine disease), hyperammonaemic syndromes (e.g. ornithine transcarbamylase deficiency) and mitochondrial disorders must be ruled out by investigation of liver function and measurement of plasma and urinary organic and amino acids, glutamine, blood ammonia after a protein-containing meal, and pyruvate and lactate after carbohydrate. Although rare, these disorders are important because they are genetically determined and some are potentially successfully treatable.

## Periodic syndrome

Cyclical episodes of malaise, pallor with dark panda-ringed eyes often with fever, nausea, vomiting and various aches also appear to be paramigrainous variants of the two foregoing conditions. They tend to occur in the age range 2–8 years. Understandably the focus of much parental anxiety, it is difficult to make a diagnosis until a cyclical pattern has been established and other more serious conditions have been ruled out. Even so, it is impossible to make a reasonably confident diagnosis of periodic syndrome except retrospectively.

## Benign paroxysmal vertigo

Benign paroxysmal vertigo is often mistaken for epileptic seizures. There is no loss of consciousness but children usually fall. Attacks last from a few seconds to several minutes and are obviously very unpleasant. The justification for considering them to be migrainous rests on the frequent coexistence of more typically migrainous symptoms during or between attacks (Dunn & Snyder 1976; Abu-Arafeh & Russell 1994).

## Benign paroxysmal torticollis

This condition, which occurs in infancy and which features episodic head tilt lasting minutes or hours, often with irritability and pallor, appears to be an infantile variant of benign paroxysmal vertigo (Dunn & Snyder 1976). The differential diagnosis includes posterior fossa space-occupying lesion. Persistent torticollis in children is more likely to signify squint or cervical dislocation.

## Benign limb pains

Pain, often awakening a child from sleep and having a very unpleasant aching quality, is very common in childhood migraine (Apley & MacKeith 1962) and is probably the basis for the lay diagnosis of 'growing pains' – a concept used to explain an essentially benign phenomenon, in contradistinction to the acute pain of rheumatism, which used to be frequent in the same age group. The mechanism is unknown and could be of central (i.e. thalamic) origin. Timing is usually completely dissociated from typical migraine attacks. Many parents believe that massage helps but aspirin is a most effective remedy, although now out of favour because of the rare hazard of precipitating Reye's syndrome in certain metabolically vulnerable children.

## Epistaxis

Recurrent epistaxis is prevalent in children with migraine and episodes may presage frankly migrainous attacks (Konomoff & Simeonoff 1968; Sperber & Arbabanel 1986). It may be a further manifestation of the vasomotor instability that has been studied in facial skin of adults with migraine and fits well with the notion that there is vasodilatation of small blood vessels which rupture easily in nasal mucosa, being relatively unsupported by connective tissue.

## Motion sickness

Motion sickness also occurs more frequently than can be due to chance in children who suffer from migraine. Acceleration, deceleration and cornering sharply are particularly provocative, presumably because of vestibular stimulation, although in some children photoresponsiveness may contribute, as in epilepsy.

## Complicated migraine – *migraine accompagnée*

As in adults, the various syndromes included under the rubric of *migraine accompagnée* are well recognised in children. These include: hemiplegic migraine; sensory migraine; basilar migraine; facioplegic migraine; ophthalmoplegic migraine; and classical migraine.

In cervical migraine, there may be accompanying neck stiffness and fever and modest CSF pleocytosis. In the most severe attacks of *migraine accompagnée* there may be permanent neurological deficits in the territory corresponding to focal symptoms or signs of the acute attack, most easily explained on a vascular basis, although a direct neuronal/chemical mechanism is also possible.

Episodic confusion, sometimes with combative behaviour followed by amnesia has been occasionally described in children as a migrainous phenomenon because of the coexistence of characteristically migrainous symptoms, although they are not invariably present (Gascon & Barlow 1970; Dinsmore & Callender 1983; D'Cruz & Walsh 1992).

Typically migrainous auras, comprising photopsias, scintillating scotomas, aberrations of perception of time or sound, but without headache, have been described in 2 per cent of children with migraine and diagnosed as 'acephalgic' migraine (Shevell 1996).

## Mechanism of attacks

Recent research in adults has dramatically advanced our understanding of the mechanism of headaches in migraine and has been succinctly reviewed elsewhere (Ferrari 1998). The initiating process is ill understood, and here only some of the predisposing and triggering factors will be explored which initiate a sequence culminating in headaches (usually) and prodromal symptoms, aura and paramigrainous phenomena (sometimes).

## Predisposing factors

### Sex

In young affected children, the sex distribution is even (Sillanpaa 1983), but from the age of 9 years, there is an increasing female preponderance, which achieves its plateau of 2:1 from 14 years onwards. Attacks also tend to be more frequent just before or at the time of menstruation.

### Inheritance

Although a family history is not invariable, a predisposition to migraine appears to be strongly inherited. Except in familial hemiplegic migraine where a locus at 19p13 has been identified (Ophoff *et al.* 1994; 1996), inheritance is likely to be polygenic.

Phenotypic variation can be readily understood as the product of the interaction between innate and exogenous factors but, if inheritance is truly polygenic, there is particularly wide scope for clinical variation. Recurrence risks are as follows (Baier & Doose 1985):

- both parents normal, one affected child        12.8 per cent
- father and one child affected                  29 per cent
- mother and one child affected                  27 per cent
- both parents and one child affected            66.7 per cent

In hemiplegic migraine dominant inheritance has long been emphasised. Single affected cases are probably more frequent but, because of biased reporting, are not readily identified as examples of hemiplegic migraine not only because of the absence of family history, but also because headache is often inconspicuous or overlooked.

In some children with mitochondrial cytopathy, migrainous headaches are prominent features but it is not known whether this is a coincidental association or not, given the frequency of migraine in children. Conversely, recent laboratory evidence of mitochondrial dysfunction has been advanced in some patients with migraine (Majamaa 1998), but as yet there is no consistent finding of matroclinal transmission in the majority of children with common migraine.

## Diet

In migraine, as in many other conditions, diet has been the focus of much interest. Although many claims are unsubstantiated, there is scientifically well-founded evidence of diet conferring a predisposition and also having a triggering effect in children with migraine and this will be discussed in greater detail below.

## Trigger factors

These include: psychological factors; physical factors, such as fatigue and extremes of temperature and climate; trauma; and diet.

## Psychological factors

Among alleged trigger factors, excitement and emotional stress are pre-eminent. The tendency of some young children to vomit and/or complain of abdominal pain in excited anticipation of, for example, a party, is well known, but school pressures are also recognised by parents as important triggers. Under this heading, the possibility of sexual abuse has also to be remembered.

The distinction between migraine and psychogenic headache in children, although sometimes blurred, is usually comparatively easy. Non-localised unvarying headaches without any associated symptoms are most likely to be psychogenic. It is not rare for typically migrainous symptoms to coexist and to be interspersed.

Discussion on the status of tension headache in children is confused by ambiguity in the meaning of 'tension' and the failure to distinguish between tension in a psychological sense, and physical tension as in the (speculative) mechanism of persistent contraction of the occipitofrontalis muscle. Until this issue is resolved, it is preferable to use the term 'psychogenic headache' where there is persuasive evidence of a psychogenic component in children whose headaches lack other specific features.

### Physical factors

Fatigue and hunger can also play a significant role. In some children coached for competitive sport or athletics whose careers have been abandoned because of troublesome migraine, it is uncertain as to whether or not it is a physically punishing training schedule or the psychological pressures of competition which is responsible. It is probable that both factors contribute.

Extremes of temperature also serve as triggers, and thundery weather conditions affect susceptible children.

### Trauma

In children, as in adults, minor head trauma may trigger attacks; some of the examples of 'concussion' described in children after minor blows to the head are probably migrainous in nature (Jan *et al.* 1997).

### Diet

In a series of over 100 children with attacks of migraine recurring at least once weekly studied by Egger *et al.* (1983) at Great Ormond Street Children's Hospital in an open trial of a few foods diet, there was reduction of 50 per cent of headaches in approximately 90 per cent of children when offending foods or drinks were excluded. In the remainder, there was evidence of sensitivity to inhaled agents such as tobacco smoke, perfume, petrol or exhaust fumes.

The second part of the trial involved a cross-over double-blind challenge in 40 children. This confirmed that the improvement seen in the open trial was not solely or even mainly a placebo response. There was a consistent reaction to foods previously identified as potential offenders in an open trial and disguised in a bland vehicle indistinguishable in appearance, taste, smell or texture from tinned placebo material for the double-blind phase of the investigation.

Over 40 provocative items were identified in the open trial. At the top of the list in order of frequency were: cow's milk, eggs, chocolate, oranges, wheat, benzoic acid, cheese, tomatoes, tartrazine and rye.

There were often multiple sensitivities, which explains why piecemeal dietary studies, excluding only one item at a time, were not usually successful in producing significant improvement.

It was impossible to identify a class of chemicals (e.g. aromatic amines) common to all provocative foods. This suggested that a direct chemical reaction was not usually involved and a delayed allergic mechanism was proposed. Neither radioallergosorbent testing (RAST) nor skin-testing was useful for identifying provocative foods, and it was concluded that the response was not immunoglobulin E (IgE)-mediated.

Although all parents identified other precipitating factors, especially psychological, these no longer served as triggers when appropriate dietary adjustment had been made, suggesting that although some foods were directly responsible for attacks, serving as triggers, in some cases, there appeared to be a threshold for headache which was exceeded only when diet and trigger acted in concert.

In the children studied at Great Ormond Street a number presented other associated clinical features suggesting a more complex condition than one involving an exclusively nocicentric mechanism. In addition to the phenomena of *migraine accompagnée,* explicable partly on the basis of local and spreading cortical inhibition, mentioned earlier, conduct disorders, especially those of the attention deficit disorder (ADD), were common. Epilepsy, focal and generalised, was encountered more frequently than could be explained by chance. Likewise rhinitis, recurrent mouth ulcers and, in girls, vaginal discharge. These phenomena, including epilepsy, improved in parallel with headaches when offending foods were excluded.

Dietary factors are also relevant in *migraine accompagnée*, including children in whom permanent deficits result from exceptionally severe attacks. The most vivid example of dietary sensitivity in *migraine accompagnée* was provided by a young child who was passionately fond of cheese but whose parents recognised that she developed headache and vomiting when any but trivial amounts were eaten. Unfortunately, while in the care of an indulgent relative who was unaware of the problem, the youngster was permitted to have approximately 250 grams of cheese with Sunday tea and within an hour became very ill with severe headache, vomiting and hemiplegia. Although there was recovery from the constitutional upset, improvement in focal weakness was incomplete.

## Investigation

The manifestations of migraine in children are protean and this obviously presents problems when other, more sinister conditions are mimicked. Diagnosis is clinical supported by exclusion of other conditions.

For children with headache as a new symptom, the overriding concern in a febrile illness is to exclude meningitis, and in a non-febrile condition to exclude raised intracranial pressure. In the former, if there is any doubt, the child should be referred for an urgent paediatric opinion, which implies ready access to facilities for lumbar puncture. In the latter, the now widespread access to brain-scanning facilities should make a diagnosis of raised intracranial pressure less inconclusive in the early stages than formerly.

**Table 10.1** Indications for further investigation of migraine

1 New symptoms or signs
2 Failure to fully recover between attacks
3 Headaches unrelieved by simple analgesics
4 Change in behaviour, personality or, in particular, school performance
5 Slowed growth or failure to thrive
6 Head circumference greater than the 98th centile or disproportionately large in comparison with parents'/siblings' head circumferences
7 Age less than 6 years
8 Vomiting prominent

*Source:* Hockaday (1990)

If headaches are worse in the morning or are associated with vomiting, there is a particular need to investigate the possibility of a space-occupying lesion, although in some children these symptoms are also characteristically migrainous features. Conversely, highly vascular cerebral tumours may present with typically migrainous symptoms.

It is equally important to consider further investigation in children with an accepted diagnosis of migraine in whom new features emerge, since they too are heirs to the same serious conditions as those to which all children are liable. Table 10.1 lists indications for further investigation.

## Management

Explanation, reassurance to parents and patient, and simple analgesia are effective in the majority of cases (Hamalainen *et al.* 1997b). In all, it is worth trying to identify offending dietary items, since their exclusion allows the possibility of cure rather than merely control.

### Prophylaxis

In evaluating the efficacy of prophylactic drugs in the management of childhood migraine, it is important to realise that there is a placebo response of at least 30 per cent, and some double-blind trials have shown a much more frequent placebo effect. Thus clonidine, for which there were sound pharmacological reasons for anticipating a favourable response, was not significantly different from placebo in double-blind trials.

For those children having severe attacks at, say, 2–4-week intervals, or more frequently, and in whom simple measures are ineffective, prophylaxis with pizotifen is helpful in many. Unfortunately, this drug is a powerful appetite stimulant and long-term weight gain is unacceptable in children, as in adults. Pizotifen may, however, be helpful in interrupting a vicious cycle of recurrent attacks, used for 2–3 months. Cyproheptadine is a similar drug which may be used as an alternative, but produces the same side-effects. Both drugs may be sedative and depressant when first introduced.

Among beta-blockers, propranolol has been shown to be of prophylactic value in double-blind trials but its use is contraindicated in children with asthma.

Anti-epileptic drugs such as phenobarbitone, phenytoin, carbamazepine and sodium valproate have been shown to be of prophylactic value in double-blind trials. The mechanism is unknown but is not thought to imply that migraine is an epileptic phenomenon, although migraine and epilepsy coexist more frequently than owing to chance.

Calcium-channel blockers such as verapamil and nifedipine can be used in children, having been shown to be of prophylactic value in adults.

The active principle in feverfew has been identified and shown to be effective in double-blind trials (Sumner *et al.* 1992; Barsby *et al.* 1993). Although cheap, the natural leaves are astringent to taste. Health shops market tableted preparations but these are not standardised satisfactorily. Nevertheless, they appeal to parents who are unhappy about using conventional pharmacopoeial preparations, and for others, they may be helpful when other remedies fail.

Acupuncture has its devotees, and techniques of biofeedback have been tried in children, apparently with success (Allen & McKeen 1991).

Among other unorthodox treatments, rose-tinted glasses have been shown to be helpful, compared with blue tints, in children with migraine (Good *et al.* 1991).

## Symptomatic treatment

In addition to simple analgesia, anxiolytic agents such as diazepam are also effective, but their use is not recommended because of problems of dependency.

The triptans, particularly sumatriptan, have been used in older children, but *ad hoc* use of medication presents problems for school-children because of the refusal of school staff to give medication when necessary and the unwillingness of head teachers to countenance children retaining their own medication. Sumatriptan is effective by injection in children, but some are very upset by the same side-effects which have troubled adults (Linder 1996). A double-blind trial of oral medication did not show significant benefit (Hamalainen *et al.* 1997a).

Ergotamine and its derivatives, though effective in children for the symptomatic treatment of attacks, do not have a regular place in management because of the practical difficulties of *ad hoc* administration in school-children. There is also the risk of ergotism in children having frequent attacks.

Methysergide is effective prophylactically, but suffers from the major disadvantage of inducing retroperitoneal and pleuro-pericardial fibrosis after prolonged use (i.e. six months or more). Its value lies in effectively breaking a vicious cycle of frequently recurring attacks. Both ergotamine and methysergide are, however, absolutely contraindicated in children and adults with *migraine accompagnée* because of the risk of inducing permanent neurological deficits or even death.

## Dietary management

Formal trials of dietary exclusion have been undertaken in children having very frequent attacks (one per week or more) but it has proved difficult to translate what was essentially a research programme to a service strategy.

The few foods diet is very restricted and unappetising and is nutritionally inadequate even with supplementation with calcium and vitamins. It comprises one meat (lamb or chicken), one carbohydrate (rice or potato), one fruit (banana or apple), one vegetable (brassica) and water. Its long-term use is unacceptable. Trial therefore has to be restricted to those children in whom attacks are occurring very frequently so that the effect of exclusion can be judged in a comparatively short time.

Partial trials with a fragmented approach are not usually successful when, as in most food-sensitive children, there are multiple offending dietary items. Nevertheless, an empirical trial excluding the commonest dietary items is worth considering.

The services of an experienced and committed dietitian are essential because of the need to translate the theory of the diet into the practice of everyday menus. Moreover, such is the complexity of manufactured foods, that a knowledgeable guide is essential to avoid unwitting exposure.

It is not known whether a dietary mechanism is relevant in the majority of patients having relatively infrequent attacks. Until there is a specific laboratory test which will identify potential sufferers and potential triggers, well-conducted trials will remain very difficult to undertake.

Starting with a partial or complete exclusion diet, if there is improvement within two weeks, excluded food can then be re-introduced successively at two-week intervals. Of course, children who have been benefited in the inaugural phases are motivated to continue a trial.

A minimum of two weeks is required to first establish benefit because in a minority of children symptoms worsen in the first few days. There are interesting analogies to phenomena of drug withdrawal and there are also similar parallels in the craving in some children for items which are provocative.

## Conclusions

The most notable difference between migraine in children and in adults is the shorter duration of attacks in children (though this may reflect difficulties and differences in assessment), and the diversity of paramigrainous phenomena. This diversity supports the view of a more extensive process than that involving the central nervous system only.

Notwithstanding the differences, there are more similarities than contrasts, and it is probable that in both children and adults, the endgame is similar. It is endgame studies which have dominated recent research into migraine in adults, and this has been both illuminating and therapeutically innovative. It has brought a dramatic, if expensive, benefit to many whose lives had been made miserable by their symptoms.

However, this approach has largely ignored mechanisms of inauguration and there is a need for identification of earlier links in the chain of pathogenesis, of which some clues have been provided by the tedious dietary research which I have described.

There have been comparatively few scientifically acceptable studies of the role of diet in adults, and much of the therapeutic initiative in this field has been seized by practitioners of complementary medicine. This is unfortunate, because the well-authenticated and scientifically rigorous studies in children have been quite wrongly dismissed owing to the prejudice which alternative medicine usually provokes among scientifically oriented doctors. I suspect that dietary research has been largely dismissed, not because it has been tried and found wanting, but because it has been found difficult and not tried (with apologies to G K Chesterton).

## *References*

Abu-Arafeh I & Russell G (1994). Prevalence of headache and migraine in childhood. *BMJ* **309**, 765–95.

Abu-Arafeh I & Russell G (1995). Prevalence and clinical features of abdominal migraine compared with those of migraine headache. *Arch Dis Child* **72**, 413–17.

Allen KD & McKeen LR (1991). Home-based multicomponent treatment of paediatric migraine. *Headache* **31**, 467–72.

Apley J & MacKeith R (1962). *The child and his symptoms*. Blackwell Scientific, Oxford, p.6.

Baier WK & Doose H (1985). Petit mal absences of childhood onset: familial prevalence of migraine and seizures. *Neuropediatrics* **16**, 84–91.

Barsby RW, Salan U, Knight DW & Hoult JR (1993). Feverfew and vascular smooth muscle: extracts from fresh and dried plants show opposing pharmacological profiles, dependent upon sesquiterpene lactone content. *Planta Medica* **59**, 20–5.

Bille B (1962). Migraine in school-children. *Acta Paed* **51** (Suppl.136), 1–151.

D'Cruz OF & Walsh DJ (1992). Acute confusional migraine: case series and review of literature (review). *Wisconsin Med J* **91**, 130–1.

Dinsmore WW & Callender ME (1983). Juvenile transient global amnesia. *J Neurol Neurosurg & Psychiat* **46**, 876–7.

Dunn DW & Snyder H (1976). Benign paroxysmal vertigo of childhood. *Amer J Dis Child* **130**, 1099–100.

Egger J, Carter CM, Wilson J, Turner MW & Soothill JF (1983). Is migraine food allergy? A double-blind controlled trial of oligoantigenic diet treatment. *Lancet* **2**, 865–9.

Ferrari MD (1998). Migraine. *Lancet* **351**, 1043–51.

Gascon G & Barlow CF (1970). Juvenile migraine presenting as an acute confusional state. *Pediatrics* **45**, 628–35.

Good PA, Taylor RH & Mortimer MJ (1991). The use of tinted glasses in childhood migraine. *Headache* **31**, 467–72.

Hamalainen ML, Hoppu K & Santavuori P (1997a). Sumatriptan for migraine attacks in children: a randomised placebo-controlled study. Do children with migraine respond to oral sumatriptan differently from adults? *Neurology* **48**, 1100–3.

Hamalainen ML, Hoppu K, Vaklkeila E & Santavuori P (1997b). Ibuprofen or acetoaminophen for the acute treatment of migraine in children or double-blind, randomized, placebo-controlled, crossover study. *Neurology* **48**, 103–7.

Hockaday JM (1990). Management of migraine. *Arch Dis Child* **65**, 1174–6.

Jan MM, Camfield PR, Gordon K & Camfield CS (1997). Vomiting after mild head injury is related to migraine. *J Pediatrics* **130**, 134–7.

Konomoff SI & Simeonoff KR (1968). Nouvelles conceptions sur l'origine diencéphalique des épistaxis et de la migraine (New concepts on the diencephalic origins of epistaxis and migraine). *Rev Neurologique* **119**, 229.

Linder SL (1996). Subcutaneous sumatriptan in the clinical setting: the first 50 consecutive patients with acute migraine in a paediatric neurology office practice. *Headache* **36**, 419–22.

Majamaa K (1998). Mitochondrial DNA haplogroup U as a risk factor for occipital stroke in migraine. *Lancet* **352**, 455–6.

Ophoff RA, van Eijk R, Sandkuijl LA, Terwindt GM, Grubben CPM, Haan J, Lindhout D, Ferrari MD & Frants RR (1994). Genetic heterogeneity of familial hemiplegic migraine. *Genomics* **22**, 21–6.

Ophoff RA, Terwindt GH, Vergouwe MN, van Eijk R, Oefner PJ, Hoffman SMG, Lamerdin JE, Mohrenweiser HW, Bulman DE, Ferrari M, Haan L, Lindhout D, van Ommen G-JB, Hofker MH, Ferrari MD & Frants RR (1996). Familial hemiplegic migraine and episodic ataxia type-2 are caused by mutations in the Ca(2+) channel gene CACNLIA4. *Cell* **87**, 543–52.

Shevell MI (1996). Acephalgic migraines of childhood. *Pediatric Neurology* **14**, 211–15.

Sillanpaa M (1983). Changes in the prevalence of migraine and other headache during the first seven school years. *Headache* **23**, 15–19.

Sillanpää M & Anttila P (1996). Increasing prevalence of headache in 7-year-old schoolchildren. *Headache* **36**, 466–70.

Sillanpää M, Piekkala P & Kero P (1991). Prevalence of head ache at preschool age in an unselected child population. *Cephalalgia* **11**, 239–41.

Sperber AD & Abarbanel JM (1986). Migraine-induced epistaxis. *Headache* **26**, 517–18.

Sumner H, Salan U, Knight DW & Hoult JR (1992). Inhibition of 5-lipoxygenase and cyclo-oxygenase in leukocytes by feverfew. Involvement of sesquiterpene lactones and other components. *Biochemical Pharmacology* **43**, 2313–20.

Symon DN & Russell G (1995). The relationship between cyclic vomiting syndrome and abdominal migraine. *J Pediat Gastroenterol Nutr* **21** (Suppl.1), 542–3.

Winner P, Martinez W, Mate L & Bello L (1995). Classification of pediatric migraine: proposed revisions to the IHS criteria. *Headache* **35**, 407–10.

Zuckerman B, Stevenson J & Bailey V (1987). Stomach aches and headaches in a community sample of pre-school children. *Pediatrics* **79**, 677–82.

Chapter 11

# The role of complementary therapies in headache treatment

*T E Whitmarsh*

## Introduction

Complementary therapies are booming across the industrialised world. In the UK, the estimated proportion of the population who has visited a practitioner of one of the main complementary therapies within the last 12 months is 7–11 per cent, representing spending of £500–1,000 million. Adding the cost of non-conventional medical products, this equates to a 1.5–3 per cent addition to the NHS annual budget funded from private means (White 1997).

Two detailed surveys have documented the extensive use of alternative medicine in the USA and its growth there (Eisenberg *et al.* 1993; 1998). 'Alternative' medicine (the term seems to be preferred in the USA to 'complementary') is functionally defined in these surveys as interventions neither taught widely at medical schools nor available at (US) hospitals. In 1990, 33 per cent of the US adult population had used at least one of 16 alternative therapies in the past year and this had increased to 42 per cent by 1997. Estimates for the total number of visits per year to alternative medicine practitioners in the USA were 427 million in 1990 and 629 million in 1997, exceeding total visits to all US primary care physicians (387 million and 385 million in 1990 and 1997 respectively). The expenditure on visits to alternative medicine practitioners in 1997 is estimated at $21.2 billion, $12.2 billion being 'out of pocket', more than the 1997 figure for out-of-pocket hospitalisations.

Alternative medicines are clearly very acceptable to many patients. In the 1997 survey (Eisenberg *et al.* 1998), nearly one in three individuals seeing a medical doctor for a condition also used some form of alternative treatment for it. Only 38 per cent discussed the alternative treatment with their physician, although the reasons for this seeming reluctance are not known. There are then many medical interventions made of which primary care practitioners are unaware and about which they have little knowledge. Purely on the grounds that many people use treatments which could have an impact on conventional care, it is reasonable to expect members of the medical profession to have at least an acquaintance with some of these techniques.

Another reason for doctors to gain some insight into complementary therapies is that some of the therapies are effective in helping patients with some conditions and appropriate delegation of care can be made with some knowledge of the likely benefits and hazards (British Medical Association 1993). There is a vital need for proper investigation in complementary medicine and it would be of enormous benefit if conventional skills in research and audit could be brought to bear on this huge area of clinical activity.

This chapter aims to provide an overview of the range and scope of complementary therapies in the care of patients presenting with headache, based mostly on the research that has been published. It does not intend to go into very much detail of the therapies and their techniques, as there are many other sources for this.

## Acupuncture

Acupuncture is probably the complementary therapy most commonly available in the UK, through its wide and increasing role in primary care, in pain clinics and in conventional physiotherapy departments. A simple MEDLINE search reveals several thousand references to acupuncture in the treatment of pain. Most of these consist of single case reports, small case series, uncontrolled studies and many theoretical papers, but meta-analyses of the effects of acupuncture in chronic pain broadly suggest that it has an effect above that of placebo in painful conditions, including headache of various forms (ter Riet *et al.* 1990; Vincent 1993).

Traditional Chinese medicine practitioners would argue that the term 'acupuncture' should be reserved for needling at points specified by traditional Chinese diagnostic techniques, guided by an appreciation of Chinese physiology and meridian theory. They would prefer so called western-style acupuncturists to use the term 'dry needling'. The majority of acupuncture performed in western cultures for painful conditions is probably based on myofascial trigger point theory (Baldry 1993), with pain being referred distantly from exquisitely tender points in musculoskeletal tissues (Figure 11.1). Dry needling of trigger points can de-activate them (Lewit 1979). There is a large literature related to peri-cranial and cervical tender points and trigger points in headache populations. For a review, see Davidoff (1998).

On the basis that de-activating trigger points reduces pain, then any patient with multiple cervical or peri-cranial trigger points should benefit from dry needling to the points. This might well include patients with cervicogenic and post-traumatic headaches, but there are no data on these issues. Most information is available about episodic and chronic tension-type headache and migraine.

A number of studies in tension-type headache have shown quite marked improvements with acupuncture. Several different trial designs have been employed, including using physiotherapy treatment as a control group (Carlsson *et al.* 1990), single-case design (Vincent 1990) and cross-over trial against placebo acupuncture (Hansen & Hansen 1985). Generally, the number of subjects has not been high (typically 10–25 patients). The difficulty of devising a convincing placebo control for acupuncture (or indeed for any physical therapy) has been much discussed (Baldry 1993). A high-quality trial of traditional Chinese acupuncture against placebo in tension-type headache assigned 30 patients to either Chinese acupuncture or a sham

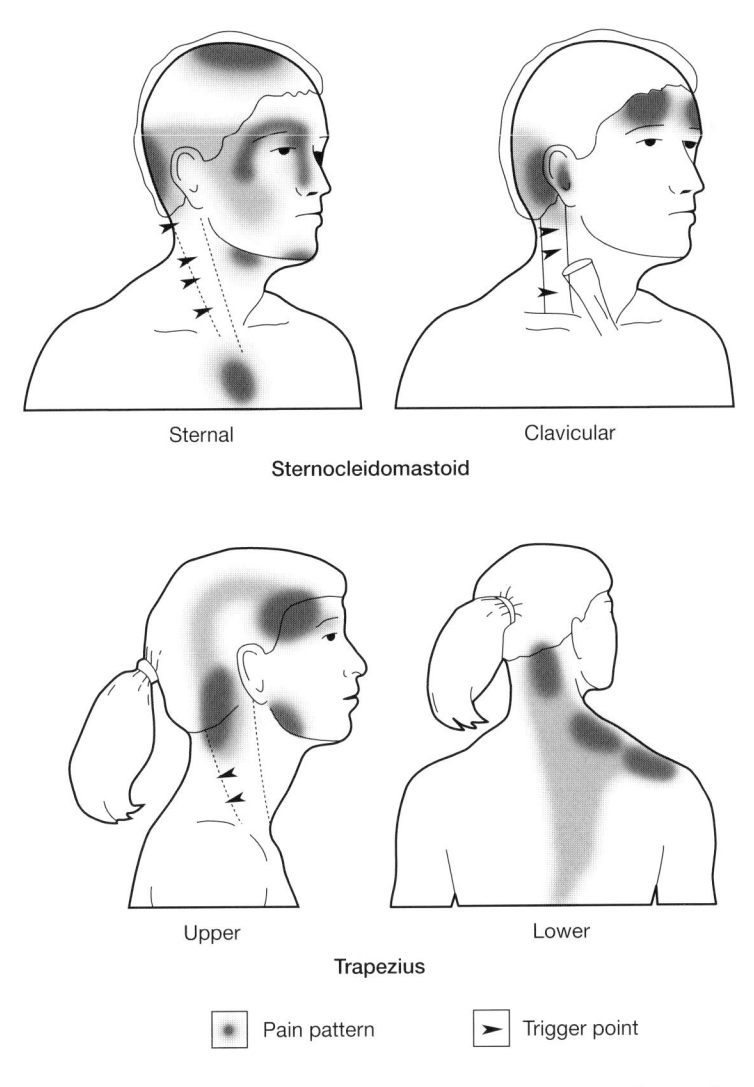

The place and efficacy of complementary therapies  **137**

**Figure 11.1** Patterns of pain referral from trigger points in two neck muscles (*Source:* Baldry 1993, p.235. Reproduced with permission)

procedure in which needles were inserted superficially a short distance away from actual points (Tavola *et al.* 1992). Both groups underwent a 20-minute session once a week for eight weeks. There were significant improvements in all measures of efficacy in both groups one month after the end of treatment, which were maintained at 12-month follow-up. There was a trend for the acupuncture group to have greater benefit, but the differences were not noteworthy. It has been suggested that the physiological effects of such a sham procedure may be not insignificant, making it more difficult to demonstrate benefits of the true procedure (Vincent 1989b). More recently, a pilot trial to investigate the credibility of a novel placebo (a cocktail stick held within a plastic guide tapped onto the skin) demonstrated an increase in headache-free weeks following a standardised acupuncture regimen encompassing treatment to trigger points in the neck compared to the sham procedure (White *et al.* 1996). The sham was also found to be credible and so may be helpful in future trials as a procedure with almost no physiological effect which should help separate out the true effects of acupuncture.

The benefits of acupuncture treatment of migraine are a little more convincing, with more controlled trials showing positive results. Once again, the control groups vary. Standard medical treatment has been used and acupuncture has been found to be of about equal prophylactic efficacy (Loh *et al.* 1984; Hesse *et al.* 1994). It is significantly more effective than sham acupuncture (Vincent 1989a; Pintov *et al.* 1997). One trial in 48 patients, using mock transcutaneous electrical nerve stimulation (TENS) as control, could only demonstrate a trend to improvement in the active group at 24-week follow-up, the advantage in reduction in mean pain scores being a non-significant 20 per cent (Dowson *et al.* 1985). A high-quality trial is that of Vincent (1989a), who randomised 30 migraine patients to true and sham acupuncture groups and demonstrated a 43 per cent reduction in weekly pain score and 38 per cent reduction in medication use at four months in the acupuncture group, compared to 14 per cent and 28 per cent reductions in pain score and medication use, respectively, in the sham group. The improvements were maintained at one-year follow-up after just six weekly treatments.

When acupuncture is effective, there can be long lasting benefits, with pain reduction being maintained for up to three years after just a few treatment sessions (Pintov *et al.* 1997). Several of the above studies also demonstrate that there are definitely a group of patients who do not respond to acupuncture, but as they cannot yet be reliably predicted, they will tend to skew the results of trials making it harder to demonstrate positive effects (Baischer 1995). The presence of depression has also been associated with relative reduction in therapeutic success in the treatment of headache by acupuncture (Klimm *et al.* 1984).

In conclusion then, it is reasonable to say that acupuncture or dry needling holds out the prospects of success in helping people with tension-type headache, particularly in the presence of active trigger points in the cervical and peri-cranial muscles. It would also appear to be at least as successful as beta-blockers in migraine prophylaxis and is a useful additional option, although it is not clear whether the presence of trigger points is always necessary for success with acupuncture in headache.

Acupuncture could be considered when medication fails or is contra-indicated, when side-effects are unbearable or when the patient declines to take long-term drugs. The effects appear to be reasonably robust and long lasting certainly in some patients, with minimal prospect of side-effects.

## Chiropractic and other manipulative therapies

In the USA, where the vast majority of chiropractic is carried out, there are an estimated 18-38 million manipulations of the cervical spine for headache each year (Shekelle & Coulter 1997). Does all this activity have an evidence base? The chiropractic literature is replete with single cases, case series and uncontrolled studies which suggest very beneficial effects of cervical spine manipulation in various forms of headache. Taking the subjects of eight case series together, 629 of 764 (82 per cent) had at least temporary improvement in their symptoms, with only 31 of 764 (4 per cent) becoming worse, 56 of 764 (7 per cent) reporting no change and 48 being unclassifiable (Hurwitz *et al.* 1996). One broad look at the literature claims between 75 and 90 per cent benefit of various forms of manipulation in headache (Vernon 1995a), but there are few trials and even fewer controlled trials. Often non-standard diagnoses have been used (for example, cervical migraine) (Stodolny & Chmielewski 1989) or only patients with 'cervical dysfunction' have been included. There does seem to be frustration in the literature at the relative lack of attention paid by conventional doctors to the role of the cervical spine in the generation and maintenance of headache. In particular, it is felt that the current model of cervicogenic headache by International Headache Society (IHS) criteria is too restrictive (International Headache Society Classification Committee 1988). Reviews by Vernon (1989; 1991; 1995a; 1995b) repeatedly complain of this, saying, for example, that 'this coherent paradigm is largely disregarded in orthodox circles' (Vernon 1995a). Quite reasonably though, chiropractors only use manipulation when there is something to treat, which will almost always be the change in the cervical spine not detectable by conventional diagnostic techniques.

What then are the headache types for which there is some evidence that chiropractic has a useful role? There are well-conducted trials with results favouring spinal manipulation over control groups in chronic tension-type headache (Boline *et al.* 1995), post-traumatic headache (Jensen *et al.* 1990), migraine (Parker *et al.* 1978; 1980) and cervicogenic headache (by IHS criteria) (Nilsson *et al.* 1997). A well-conducted study in episodic tension-type headache showed no specific benefit of spinal manipulation (Bove & Nilsson 1998). There are, of course, similar problems of defining an adequate control procedure for manipulative therapies as there are with trials of acupuncture. Double-blinding of these trials is not possible: they have to be single-blind or open, with all the confounding variables and the inevitable debate about the contribution of the placebo effect to any results.

The best randomised controlled trial of chiropractic in chronic tension-type headache, diagnosed by IHS criteria, is that of Boline (1995). One hundred and twenty-six patients were randomised to either chiropractic spinal manipulation or to standard drug therapy with low-dose amitriptyline. The chiropractic group (n=70) received 20 minutes of treatment twice a week for six weeks and the amitriptyline group (n=56) received 10-30 mg of amitriptyline daily for six weeks. Both groups improved at similar rates during the treatment period in all outcome measures. Four weeks after the end of the intervention, however, the spinal manipulation group showed a 32 per cent reduction in headache intensity, 42 per cent in headache frequency, 30 per cent in over-the-counter medication usage and 16 per cent improvement in functional health status (assessed by SF-36) in relation to the baseline values. All differences were statistically significant (p≤.008) in favour of the manipulation group. The amitriptyline therapy group showed no improvement over baseline values at four weeks post-treatment. Of course, many questions can be asked about the reliability of these results, in particular the fact that no placebo group was used and that follow-up was relatively short. Conclusions cannot therefore be definitively drawn about whether spinal manipulation provided therapeutic benefit beyond that of placebo. The choice of the intervention generally held to be effective and shown to be so in some placebo-controlled trials as the control condition – drug therapy with amitriptyline – makes this conclusion more likely, as does the sustained benefit in the manipulation group following cessation of therapy.

Jensen *et al.* (1990) studied post-traumatic headache and compared 'manual therapy', a form of osteopathic manipulation, with the application of cold packs to the neck as a control group. This was a small study, with ten patients in the manual therapy group and nine in the cold-pack group. The intervention was minimal with only two treatments of each form of therapy, but the mean pain index was significantly reduced to 43 per cent of baseline in the group treated with manual therapy compared with the cold-pack group. Five-week follow-up showed that the pain index was still lower in the manual therapy group compared to the cold-pack group, although the difference was no longer significant. Patients were not categorised by IHS criteria. Although the study is small and beneficial result not sustained, the intervention was extremely minimal and does not conform to usual general osteopathic practice. One might expect more sustained improvement with more frequent therapy sessions.

The only randomised controlled trial of spinal manipulation in migraine (Parker *et al.* 1978; 1980) compared chiropractic manipulation (n=30), manipulation given by a medical doctor (n=27) and mobilisation by physiotherapists (n=28). The chiropractic group had a greater reduction in frequency of attacks after two months' treatment (mean 7 sessions), although it did not reach statistical significance and a significant reduction in severity of attacks compared to the other groups. At 20-month follow-up, the chiropractic patients had significantly fewer attacks.

A well-performed study in cervicogenic headache, diagnosed by IHS criteria (Nilsson *et al.* 1997), randomised 53 subjects into receiving either cervical manipulation or low-level laser treatment and deep friction massage in the lower cervical and upper thoracic regions. These interventions were performed twice a week for three weeks. The low-energy laser can be expected to have an effect equivalent to placebo and was used to provide another form of cervical intervention, making the groups as similar as possible. Comparing a baseline week to the week after the intervention was finished, the use of analgesics, the number of headache hours per day and the headache intensity per episode all decreased significantly in the manipulation group compared to the control group. It can be reasonably concluded that spinal manipulation has a positive effect in cervicogenic headache.

The same group recently published a trial of the same methodology in 75 patients with episodic tension-type headache (Bove & Nilsson 1998). The trial ran for 19 weeks and all participants received eight treatments over four weeks after a baseline two weeks. By week 7, both groups had experienced significant reductions in mean daily headache hours and mean number of analgesics used per day and these benefits were maintained through the trial with no differences between groups. The headache pain intensity was unchanged for the duration of the trial. Spinal manipulation, isolated from any other intervention, does not appear to be effective in episodic tension-type headache.

These last two well-conducted trials used identical methodology and demonstrate how important it is to differentiate types of headache which may respond to a manipulative intervention. In the second paper the authors make the point that episodic tension-type headache and cervicogenic headache often occur together and may be very difficult to differentiate. How is the non-specialised manipulator to decide when referral for physical therapy to the neck is appropriate? An attempt to answer this has been made in an interesting systematic review of cervical spine manipulation (Hurwitz *et al.* 1996) and a subsequent multidisciplinary expert panel (Shekelle & Coulter 1997). Based on the systematic review, a summary was sent to nine experts in the field of cervical spine manipulation and headache, including an orthopaedic surgeon, a neurosurgeon, two neurologists, a primary care physician and four chiropractors.

The panel members then used a risk-benefit scale to rate for appropriateness the use of cervical spine manipulation in a wide-ranging list of 736 clinically detailed presentation scenarios. Their opinions were collated and a conference was held with discussion of the contentious points. After discussion they re-rated each scenario, judging 82 as appropriate, 230 as uncertain, and 424 as inappropriate for cervical spine manipulation. Their judgement of clinical features which are most associated with indications for patients with headache being rated as appropriate for cervical spine manipulation are reproduced in Table 11.1. They give an idea of the kind of patients who might benefit from referral to a chiropractor or other manipulative therapist and perhaps represent a first attempt at some guidelines.

Chiropractic is not without its risks, although these are very small. The review of Hurwitz *et al.* (1996) identified 136 references to complications of cervical spine manipulation in the literature from 1966 to 1996. Twenty-three of these occurred when headache was the presenting complaint, but serious complications of cervical spine manipulation have a very low incidence of between 10 and 20 per 10 million manipulations.

**Table 11.1** Clinical characteristics of headache patients most likely to benefit from spinal manipulative therapy (SMT)

*Acute constant headache (<3 weeks in duration)*

- History of related cervical spine trauma
- No post-traumatic neurologic symptoms
- No radiographic contraindications to SMT
- No neurologic findings
- Presence of cervical signs or symptoms
- Non-manipulative conservative care for this episode has failed
- Prior favourable response to SMT

*Acute or subacute intermittent headache (<3 months in duration)*

- No radiographic contraindications to SMT
- No neurologic symptoms or findings
- Presence of cervical signs or symptoms
- Prior favourable response to SMT
- If no prior SMT, add no history of related cervical spine trauma

*Chronic intermittent headache (>3 months' duration)*

- Non-throbbing with no prodrome
    - No clinical risk factors or no radiographic contraindications to SMT
    - Presence of cervical signs or symptoms
    - No prior SMT or prior favourable response to SMT
- With throbbing or prodrome
    - No clinical risk factors or no radiographic contraindications to SMT
    - Presence of cervical signs or symptoms
    - Prior favourable response to SMT

*Source:* Shekelle & Coulter (1997), p.226. Reproduced with permission

All in all then, the literature is very incomplete, with the most exhaustive systematic review (Hurwitz *et al.* 1996) being able to go no further than stating that manipulation and/or mobilisation may be beneficial for tension-type headache. The uptake of cervical manipulation, however, belies the literature. A comparison of more specialised techniques with more generally available physiotherapy techniques would be extremely interesting.

## Homeopathy

In a thorough meta-analysis of clinical trials of homeopathy (Linde *et al.* 1997) the hypothesis that the effects seen with homeopathic remedies are equivalent to those with placebo was tested. By diligent searching, 189 randomised and blinded placebo controlled trials were identified and 119 met the entry criteria, with 89 having adequate data for meta-analysis. The combined odds ratio for the 89 studies was 2.45 (95 per cent confidence intervals 2.052–2.93). Corrections for study quality and for possible publication bias made little difference to the conclusion that there is no evidence to suggest that the clinical effects of homeopathy are completely due to placebo. Two other meta-analyses, using different methods, reached broadly similar conclusions (Kleijnen *et al.* 1991; Boissel *et al.* 1996).

Homeopathy has long been acclaimed as effective in the treatment of migraine and other headaches (Cooper 1984). There are single-case reports of extreme effectiveness in some patients (Reilly 1990; Whitmarsh 1997) and one double-blind placebo-controlled trial showing highly significant reductions in all parameters of headache in a population of 60 migraine sufferers (Brigo & Serpelloni 1991).

The question of reproducibility of results of clinical trials is central to the credibility of therapeutic interventions. The literature on complementary therapies is particularly deficient with regard to repetitions of studies using similar methodology and similar outcome measures in similar populations. Trials of homeopathy in headache exemplify the problems.

An attempt was made by Whitmarsh *et al.* (1997) to reproduce the results of the earlier study. In Brigo's study, it is unlikely that all cases included would meet the IHS criteria for diagnosis, and certainly trial design recommendations (International Headache Society Committee on Clinical Trials in Migraine 1991) were not followed, since it was conducted before these were available. This second study incorporated a number of quality criteria, including the use of IHS classification and trial design recommendations, an explicit primary outcome measure (headache frequency per month) and good clinical practice (GCP) monitoring. Sixty patients were randomised to active homeopathy or placebo groups and treated for three months after a baseline one-month run-in. The attack frequency declined in both groups, by 16 per cent in those treated with placebo and 19 per cent in those who received homeopathy, an insignificant difference (Figure 11.2).

Although the primary outcome measure was not particularly influenced by homeopathy at the end of the treatment period, the course of change was different in the two groups. Improvement occurred early in the placebo group, followed by a return towards baseline by the end of the trial. By contrast, the active group improved later and was still continuing its improvement when the trial ended, and the authors regret that the study period, chosen according to IHS recommendations, was not longer, to allow any difference over time to appear. Homeopathic physicians frequently observe long-lasting, but slow onset effects of treatment (Boyd 1989).

Furthermore, after randomisation, there was a chance difference between groups for both the primary outcome measure and also for headache severity, with the placebo group having more frequent but less severe headaches. Closer analysis revealed that the homeopathically treated group lost their moderate-to-severe headaches,

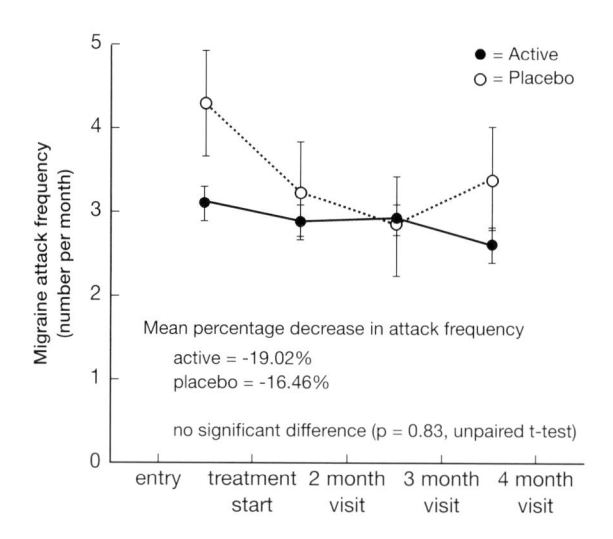

**Figure 11.2** Homoeopathic prophylaxis of migraine. Change in mean attack frequency per month by treatment group (active versus placebo) during the trial. Bars represent standard deviations. The groups were not well matched at entry. Each group showed a small improvement, and these appeared to follow different courses; early on placebo, later on homoeopathy. There was a suggestion that, as follow-up ended, the effect of placebo, but not of homoeopathy, was undergoing reversal (*Source*: Whitmarsh *et al.* 1997, p.603. Reproduced with permission)

whereas the placebo group lost their mild headaches only. Attack frequency thus was relatively stable over the short treatment period, but headache severity may have changed significantly.

A third large randomised double-blind trial of homeopathy in chronic headache, most cases of which suffered migraine or tension-type headache by IHS criteria, was reported by Walach *et al.* (1997). Sixty-one patients received individualised homeopathic treatment and 37 received placebo. The trial quality was high with a six-week baseline observation period and 12 weeks of treatment. Data were entered daily in diaries, with headache intensity recorded on a visual analogue scale. Patients improved a little in both groups, but there were no significant differences in any measure of outcome between the groups. These patients were a difficult group to help by any standards, with a median headache frequency of three days per week and a median duration of symptoms of 23 years. Initial interview was by one of six homeopathic doctors, who discussed each case with all their colleagues before prescribing and spent a mean of 156 minutes on the case-taking. This method of prescribing and a long first interview do not correspond to the usual practice of the majority of homeopathic physicians.

A Norwegian study of 68 patients with IHS-diagnosed migraine and a four-month follow-up period with active homeopathy compared to placebo (Straumsheim *et al.* 1997) showed a significant reduction in headache frequency in the active group (60 per cent decline in active group, against 42 per cent in the placebo group, p=0.04). This difference was, however, only demonstrated with an independent neurologist's assessment, not from patient self-reports.

The startling levels of significance in all headache parameters seen in the first trial (Brigo & Serpelloni 1991) were therefore nowhere replicated in these studies, but it would be wrong to lump all of the trials together and conclude that homeopathy on the whole has no activity in migraine above that of placebo: the trials are not comparable in study populations, diagnostic criteria, methodology or outcome measures. Despite the confusion of these trials, homeopathic physicians continue to be quite confident in prescribing for migraine and headache (Boyd 1989; Whitmarsh 1997). These observations raise questions about applicability of conventional trial design to complementary therapies and the kind of outcome measures which could make a convincing case for changes in the practice of both complementary practitioners and conventional physicians.

## Food intolerance and dietary supplements

Many foods have been reported to idiosyncratically precipitate attacks of migraine (Peatfield *et al.* 1984) and most physicians routinely search for possible trigger factors of migraine, including dietary ones and counsel avoidance. The idea of migraine as a food-allergic disorder has also been often raised (Grant 1979). Evidence for this comes from noticeable improvements in headache frequency and/or severity after exclusion of various foods from the diet, followed by double-blind placebo-controlled re-introductions of specific food triggers in paediatric (Egger *et al.* 1983) and adult (Cornwell & Clarke 1991) sufferers. In the paediatric study, 85 per cent of 98 migraine sufferers became headache-free after following an elimination diet for four weeks. Sixty responders were then challenged in a double-blind trial with the offending foods and only redeveloped migraine with the true foods but not with sham foods. Correlations of food-induced migraine with specific immunoglobulin E to the foods implicated by dietary exclusion (by radioallergosorbent testing) (Munro *et al.* 1980) and with skin testing to dietary allergens (Mansfield *et al.* 1985) have been observed. A protective effect of sodium cromoglycate has also been noted (Munro *et al.* 1984). Little has been published about food allergy in migraine since a flurry of activity in the early 1980s, but the lines of research suggested then are still of great interest. If disabling migraine can truly be managed by (admittedly, at times rather tricky) dietary means, then they are surely worth including in the armamentarium of migraine prophylaxis.

Recently, there has been interest in the role of magnesium in migraine (Mauskop & Altura 1998). Prompted by observations of low magnesium levels in various body tissues of migraine sufferers and by the fact that magnesium deficiency has wide-ranging physiological effects, one trial randomised 81 migraine patients to oral magnesium dicitrate 600 mg (24 mmol) for 12 weeks or to placebo (Peikert *et al.* 1996). Within weeks 9–12, attack frequency was reduced by 41 per cent in the magnesium group and by 15.8 per cent in the placebo group compared to the baseline (p<0.05).

Another small trial in menstrual migraine had similarly positive results (Facchinetti *et al.* 1991) but a further carefully conducted study was terminated because of lack of efficacy of 20 mmol of magnesium against placebo at an interim analysis of 69 patients (Pfaffenrath *et al.* 1996). The authors admit to potential biases in the study and recommend further investigation perhaps with higher doses and a new design.

Mauskop has observed in acute migraine (Mauskop *et al.* 1995a) and cluster headache (Mauskop *et al.* 1995b) attacks that patients with low serum ionised magnesium levels respond to intravenous infusion of magnesium sulphate. The results are impressive with, for example in migraine, a pain reduction of 50 per cent or more within 15 minutes of infusion in 35 acute attacks, with significantly more patients responding if their serum ionised magnesium levels were low. These results, however, have not yet been subjected to double-blind controlled assessment.

Another substance which might be thought of as a food supplement is riboflavin (vitamin $B_2$). On the grounds of a possible mitochondrial oxidative phosphorylation defect suggested by magnetic spectroscopy of the brain during migraine attacks, Schoenen *et al.* (1994) suggested its use in migraine. Riboflavin is a precursor of the co-enzymes flavin mononucleotide and flavin adenine dinucleotide, which are required in oxidation-reduction reactions. There has been beneficial clinical response in various mitochondrial myopathies to riboflavin. An open prophylactic study of high-dose riboflavin (400 mg daily) in 49 migraineurs for three months resulted in 'global improvement' of 82 per cent (Schoenen *et al.* 1994). A randomised double-blind placebo-controlled trial followed, with 55 patients randomised to 400mg riboflavin or placebo daily (Schoenen *et al.* 1998). After three months of treatment, the mean number of migraine attacks per month in the riboflavin group decreased from 3.83 to less than 2 (p = .0001). There was a parallel decrease in the number of days of migraine and the duration of the headache. There were no changes in the placebo group (Figure 11.3). The number needed to treat for a 50 per cent reduction in attack frequency was 2.8, and 2.3 for a 50 per cent reduction in headache days. Adverse events were minimal with only one riboflavin recipient leaving the study after two weeks because of diarrhoea.

Riboflavin in high dose (at least 20 times the recommended daily intake) would appear on this evidence to be a useful option for migraine prophylaxis, but of course further work needs to be done, particularly with trials against more conventional prophylactic agents.

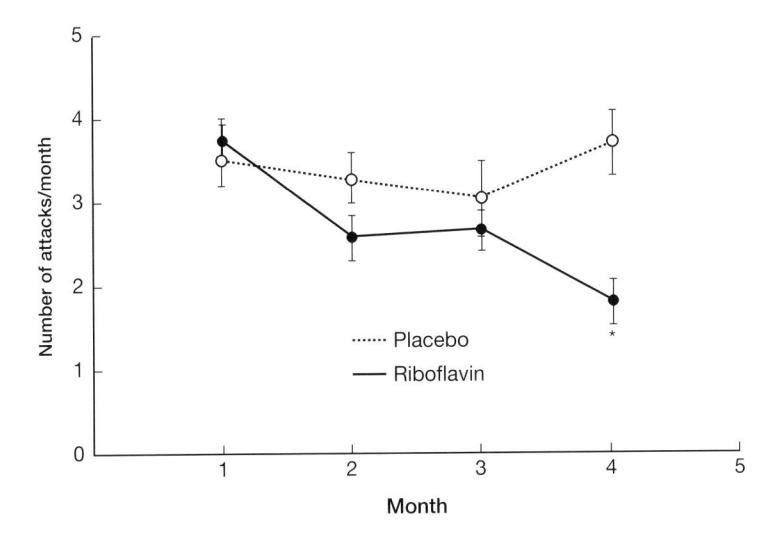

**Figure 11.3** Mean number of migraine attacks per month during the 4-month trial in placebo (n=26) and riboflavin 400mg groups (n=28). Compared with baseline (placebo) month 1, the decrease of attack frequency becomes significant in the riboflavin group during month 4 (*p=0.0001), which is the third month of the randomised phase (*Source*: Schoenen *et al.* 1998, p.468. Reproduced with permission)

In summary it seems that there is a definite group of migraine sufferers who can be headache-free if they can avoid triggering foods and it is reasonable to help them identify these. There may be a role of the immune system, with food sensitivity being reasonably well established in some groups, particularly children, but again more work needs to be done here before sure conclusions can be reached and treatment guidelines drawn up. Magnesium and especially vitamin $B_2$ in daily high dosages are genuine practical additions to the range of treatments available for migraine prophylaxis. They are cheap and have an excellent tolerability and side-effect profile. Whether their action will enhance the value of other prophylactic measures remains to be seen.

## Biobehavioural techniques

A number of these 'calming' techniques are in widespread use for the treatment of headache, mostly with prophylactic intent. They include biofeedback, relaxation, autogenic training, hypnosis and meditation (Reid & McGrath 1996; Van Hook 1998).

Biofeedback is the use of electronic displays to collect and show physiological processes to the patient, with the goal of increasing the patient's control over the internal processes and changing them at will. There are many different forms of biofeedback, but the more frequently used and studied are thermal biofeedback and electromyogram (EMG) biofeedback. In the former, the patient attempts to raise the temperature of a finger and, in the latter, the patient aims to change the activity of muscles measured by EMG electrodes, usually placed, in headache treatment, on muscles of the head and neck. The literature on biofeedback as treatment for headache is extensive, most of it emanating from North America, where it is standard practice in many headache treatment centres and hardly deserves the title 'complementary' in this context. It is not, however, commonly employed in the UK.

Studies suggest that biofeedback is effective in the prophylaxis of migraine (Grazzi & Bussone 1993) and tension-type headache (Chapman 1986; Bogaards & ter Kuile 1994) and that its effects are prolonged (Gauthier & Carrier 1991). One review of 25 controlled studies in migraine suggests comparable efficacy to standard prophylactic drug treatment (Holroyd & Penzien 1990), although it is, at least initially, much more time-consuming. There may be some advantage in combining biofeedback with other calming techniques (Hermann *et al.* 1995). Successful biofeedback appears to induce the state of deep relaxation.

Relaxation, of course, can be achieved without electronic feedback – the two most widely taught forms of relaxation training being progressive muscular relaxation and autogenic training. Autogenic training has frequently been studied in chronic headache patients and found to be effective (ter Kuile *et al.* 1994). It consists of a series of easily learned mental exercises which aim to link mind and body together in association with deep relaxation. The technique can be learned with weekly sessions over 8–10 weeks. Skills learned in the training are adaptable to any life situation and have the effect of reducing stress responses.

Hypnotherapy has been found to be effective, mostly in uncontrolled studies, in tension-type headache (VanDick *et al.* 1991) and migraine (Anderson *et al.* 1975). A literature review of 26 articles (Primavera & Kaiser 1992) could find no significant difference in overall efficacy of hypnosis, biofeedback and relaxation training. In addition, very few factors have been demonstrated to predict which patients will respond to which technique (ter Kuile *et al.* 1995), although, perhaps not surprisingly, there is evidence that hypnotisability does predict positive outcome with hypnosis and autogenic training (ter Kuile *et al.* 1994).

Biofeedback and relaxation should probably be more generally available particularly for management of resistant migraine and chronic tension-type headache. The use of hypnotherapy is perhaps best reserved for those who state a strong preference, but it seems as though any form of therapy which can induce a relaxation response has a beneficial effect on headache sufferers. There are case reports of extremely effective relief of chronic headache with the technique of transcendental meditation (Lovell-Smith 1985). Again, for highly motivated patients this may be a good option.

## Feverfew

No discussion of complementary treatments of migraine is complete without consideration of the herb feverfew (*Tanacetum parthenium*). It has been recommended for centuries for the treatment of many different symptoms, particularly for headache and latterly migraine (Heptinstall 1988). The original double-blind study examined the effects of withdrawal of feverfew from regular users and demonstrated a significant deterioration in migraine in those changed to placebo, but the patients were self-selected and the results could not be generalised (Johnson et al. 1985). A later prospective double-blind cross-over placebo-controlled trial randomised 72 patients to receive either one capsule of dried feverfew leaves a day or matching placebo for four months (Murphy et al. 1988). The patients then transferred to the other treatment arm for another four months. Treatment with feverfew reduced the frequency and severity of attacks and the amount of vomiting to a significant degree. There were mild, insignificant side-effects.

Three further double-blind studies (Kuritzky et al. 1994; DeWeert et al. 1996; Pavlevitch et al. 1997) and a systematic review of all five trials (Vogler et al. 1998) have now appeared. The data on a total of 216 patients favour feverfew over placebo in the prophylaxis of migraine, though the authors of the review do have several caveats relating to the quality of the studies, which prevent them from drawing firm conclusions. On the whole, though, feverfew does appear to be a moderately effective migraine prophylactic agent with a good safety profile and tolerability. It is certainly likely to be attractive to some groups of patients. Herbalists see feverfew as a 'warming herb' and one author suggests that it should be useful in those migraine patients who gain some relief with the use of a hot pack to the head (Mills 1991).

## Other therapies
### Aromatherapy

The application of aromatic essential oils to the skin of the head and neck is widely recommended and practised for the relief of headache (Tisserand 1985). One study looked at the effects of essential oil application on a battery of neuro-psychological, physiological and pain parameters in 32 healthy subjects (Gobel et al. 1994). There were significant effects of the combination of peppermint oil, eucalyptus oil and ethanol, with an increase in cognitive performance and a muscle-relaxing and mind-relaxing effect, although pain sensitivity was not changed. Peppermint oil and ethanol did produce an analgesic effect with a reduction in sensitivity to headache. Aromatherapy has not been tested in a formal clinical trial of headache sufferers, but the observations of effects on physiological parameters which are associated with the pathophysiology of headache are of great interest as a start in the validation of such widespread empirical use.

### Alexander Technique

This is a form of postural re-integration and education which places particular emphasis on the relationship between the head and the neck. It is claimed to be effective in some patients with migraine (Barlow 1973). Anecdotally, it has a particular role in highly motivated patients who are more comfortable with self-help techniques than with manipulative or drug therapy.

## Cranial osteopathy

Cranial osteopathy (or cranio-sacral therapy) evolved from the osteopathic tradition and relies on an observation that there is a slight mobility of the skull sutures even in the adult. The cranial osteopath manipulates the skull bones in accordance with the rhythmical breathing patterns and pressure changes which results from this. It would seem to have particular applicability to post-head injury problems. Again, this contention relies purely on anecdote, as there are no study reports.

## Conclusions

This overview has aimed to inform about the range of non-conventional therapies and the various levels of evidence that exist for their efficacy in headache, from the point of view of a physician with daily experience of complementary therapies and their use in an integrative fashion with more usual treatments. The Canadian Headache Society has produced an impressive set of guidelines for the non-pharmacological management of migraine generated from a literature review and a consensus conference, which expresses the views of a group of neurologists (Pryse-Phillips *et al.* 1998).

Many headache sufferers are using the treatments discussed here either as their complete symptom management strategy, or as complementary add-on therapy to more conventional techniques. It seems reasonable that physicians dealing with headache patients should be aware of at least the outline characteristics of the most widely used complementary therapies. More detailed consideration of the literature, such as that presented here, might lead some to direct their patients toward appropriate non-conventional interventions, with reasonable expectation of beneficial outcome. Complementary medicine is at a very early stage of building up its evidence base and there remains an immense amount of work to do, but the initial pointers look promising.

*Acknowledgements*

With grateful thanks to Mary Gooch and Sandra Davies of The British Homoeopathic Library, Glasgow Homoeopathic Hospital, for literature searching, and to Janet Alexander for secretarial support.

## *References*

Anderson J A D, Bastian M A & Dalton R (1975). Migraine and hypnotherapy. *Int J Clin Exp Hypn* **23**, 48–58.

Baischer W (1995). Acupuncture in migraine: long-term outcome and predicting factors. *Headache* **35**, 472–4.

Baldry P E (1993). *Acupuncture, trigger points and musculoskeletal pain*. Churchill Livingstone, Edinburgh.

Barlow W (1973). *The Alexander principle*. Gollancz, London.

Bogaards M C & ter Kuile M M (1994). Treatment of recurrent tension headache: a meta-analytic review. *Clin J Pain* **10**, 174–90.

Boissel JP, Cucherat M, Haugh M & Gauthier E (1996). *Critical literature review of the effectiveness of homoeopathy: overview of data from homoeopathic medicine trials.* Homoeopathic Medicine Research Group. Report to the European Commission. Brussels, pp.195–210.

Boline P D, Kassak K, Bronfort G, Nelson C & Anderson A V (1995). Spinal manipulation vs. amitriptyline for the treatment of chronic tension-type headaches: a randomised clinical trial. *J Manipulative Physiol Ther* **18**, 148–54.

Bove D C & Nilsson N (1998). Spinal manipulation in the treatment of episodic tension-type headache. A randomised controlled trial. *JAMA* **280**, 1576–9.

Boyd H (1989). *Introduction to homoeopathic medicine.* Beaconsfield Publishers, Beaconsfield.

Brigo B & Serpelloni G (1991). Homoeopathic treatment of migraine: a randomised, double-blind controlled study of 60 cases (homoeopathy v placebo). *Berl J Res Hom* **1**, 98–106.

British Medical Association (1993). *Complementary medicine. New approaches to good practice.* Oxford University Press, Oxford.

Carlsson J, Fahlcrantz A & Augustinsson L-E (1990). Muscle tenderness in tension headache treated with acupuncture or physiotherapy. *Cephalalgia* **10**, 131–41.

Chapman S L (1986). A review and clinical perspective on the use of EMG and thermal biofeedback for chronic headaches. *Pain* **27**, 1–43.

Cooper D (1984). Migraine: a homoeopathic approach. *Br Hom J* **73**, 1–10.

Cornwell N & Clarke L (1991). Dietary modification in patients with migraine and tension-type headache. *Cephalalgia* **11** (Suppl.11), 143–4.

Davidoff R A (1998). Trigger points and myofascial pain: toward understanding how they affect headaches. *Cephalalgia* **18**, 436–48.

DeWeert C J, Bootsma H P R & Hendriks H (1996). Herbal medicines in migraine prevention: randomised double-blind placebo-controlled cross-over trial of a feverfew preparation. *Phyto-medicine* **3**, 225–30.

Dowson D I, Lewith G T & Machin D (1985). The effects of acupuncture versus placebo in the treatment of headache. *Pain* **21**, 35–42.

Egger J, Wilson J, Carter C M, Turner M W & Soothill J F (1983). Is migraine food allergy? A double-blind controlled trial of oligoantigenic diet treatment. *Lancet* **2**, 865–9.

Eisenberg D M, Kessler R C, Foster C *et al.* (1993). Unconventional medicine in the United States. *N Engl J Med* **328**, 246–52.

Eisenberg D M, Davis R B, Ettner S L *et al.* (1998). Trends in alternative medicine use in the United States, 1990–1997. *JAMA* **280**, 1569–74.

Facchinetti F, Sauces G, Borella P, Genazzani A R & Nappi G (1991). Magnesium prophylaxis of menstrual migraine: effects on intracellular magnesium. *Headache* **31**, 298–301.

Gauthier J G & Carrier S (1991). Longterm effects of biofeedback on migraine headache: a prospective follow-up study. *Headache* **31**, 605–12.

Gobel H, Schmidt G & Soyka D (1994). Effect of peppermint and eucalyptus oil preparations on neurophysiological and experimental algesimetric headache parameters. *Cephalalgia* **14**, 228–34.

Grant E C G (1979). Food allergies and migraine. *Lancet* **2**, 966–8.

Grazzi L & Bussone G (1993). Italian experience of electromyographic treatment of episodic common migraine: preliminary results. *Headache* **33**, 439–41.

Hansen P E & Hansen J H (1985). Acupuncture treatment of chronic tension headache – a controlled cross-over trial. *Cephalalgia* **5**, 137–42.

Heptinstall S (1988). Feverfew – an ancient remedy for modern times? *J Roy Soc Med* **81**, 373–4.

Hermann C, Kim M & Blanchard E B (1995). Behavioural and prophylactic pharmacological intervention studies of pediatric migraine: an exploratory meta-analysis. *Pain* **60**, 239–56.

Hesse J, Mogelvang B & Simonsen H (1994). Acupuncture versus metoprolol in migraine prophylaxis: a randomised trial of trigger point inactivation. *J Int Med* **235**, 451–6.

Holroyd K A & Penzien D B (1990). Pharmacological versus non-pharmacological prophylaxis of recurrent migraine headache: a meta-analytic review of clinical trials. *Pain* **42**, 1–13.

Hurwitz E L, Aker P D, Adams A H, Meeker W C & Shekelle P G (1996). Manipulation and mobilisation of the cervical spine. A systematic review of the literature. *Spine* **21**, 1746–60.

International Headache Society Classification Committee (1988). Classification and diagnostic criteria for headache disorders, cranial neuralgias and facial pain. *Cephalalgia* **8** (Suppl.7), 13–96.

International Headache Society Committee on Clinical Trials in Migraine (1991). Guidelines for controlled trials of drugs in migraine. 1st edn. *Cephalalgia* **11**, 1–12.

Jensen O K, Nielsen F F & Vosmar L (1990). An open study comparing manual therapy with use of cold packs in the treatment of post-traumatic headache. *Cephalalgia* **10**, 241–50.

Johnson E S, Kadan N P, Hylands D M & Hylands P J (1985). Efficacy of feverfew as prophylactic treatment of migraine. *Br Med J* **291**, 569–73.

Kleijnen J, Knipschild P & ter Riet G (1991). Clinical trials of homoeopathy. *Br Med J* **302**, 316–23.

Klimm J, Klimczyk R & Penninger M (1984). Effect of acupuncture in chronic headache depending on depression. *Pain* (Suppl.2), S152.

Kuritzky A, Elhachan Y, Yerushalmi Z & Hering R (1994). Feverfew in the treatment of migraine: its effect on serotonin uptake and platelet activity. *Neurology* **44** (Suppl.2), 293P.

Lewit K (1979). The needle effect in the relief of myofascial pain. *Pain* **6**, 83–90.

Linde K, Clausius N, Ramirez G *et al.* (1997). Are the clinical effects of homoeopathy placebo effects? A meta-analysis of placebo-controlled trials. *Lancet* **350**, 834–43.

Loh L, Nathan P W, Schott G D & Zilkha K J (1984). Acupuncture versus medical treatment for migraine and muscle tension headaches. *J Neurol Neurosurg Psych* **47**, 333–7.

Lovell-Smith H D (1985). Transcendental meditation and three cases of migraine. *NZ Med J* **98**, 443–5.

Mansfield L E, Vaughan T R, Waller S F, Haverly R W & Ting S (1985). Food allergy and migraine, double-blind and mediator confirmation of an allergic etiology. *Ann Allergy* **55**, 126–9.

Mauskop A & Altura B M (1998). Role of magnesium in the pathogenesis and treatment of migraines. *Clin Neurosci* **5**, 24–7.

Mauskop A, Altura B T, Cracco R Q & Altura B M (1995a). Intravenous magnesium sulphate relieves migraine attacks in patients with low serum ionised magnesium levels: a pilot study. *Clin Sci* **89**, 633–6.

Mauskop A, Altura B T, Cracco R Q & Altura B M (1995b). Intravenous magnesium sulphate relieves cluster headaches in patients with low serum ionised magnesium levels. *Headache* **35**, 597–600.

Mills S Y (1991). *The essential book of herbal medicine*. Penguin Books, London.

Munro J, Carini C, Brostoff J & Zilkha K (1980). Food allergy in migraine. Study of dietary exclusion and RAST. *Lancet* **2**, 1–4.

Munro J, Carini C & Brostoff J (1984). Migraine is a food-allergic disease. *Lancet* **2**, 719–21.

Murphy J J, Heptinstall S & Mitchell J R A (1988). Randomised placebo-controlled trial of feverfew in migraine prevention. *Lancet* **2**, 189–92.

Nilsson N, Christensen H W & Hartvigsen J (1997). The effect of spinal manipulation in the treatment of cervicogenic headache. *J Manipulative Physiol Ther* **20**, 326–30.

Parker G B, Tupling H & Pryor D S (1978). A controlled trial of cervical manipulation for migraine. *Aust NZ J Med* **8**, 589–93.

Parker G B, Pryor D S & Tupling H (1980). Why does migraine improve during a clinical trial? Further results from a trial of cervical manipulation for migraine. *Aust NZ J Med* **10**, 192–8.

Pavlevitch D, Earon G & Carasso R (1997). Feverfew as a prophylactic treatment for migraine: a double-blind placebo-controlled study. *Phytother Res* **11**, 508–11.

Peatfield R C, Glover V, Littlewood J T, Sandler M & Clifford Rose F (1984). The prevalence of diet-induced migraine. *Cephalalgia* **4**, 179–83.

Peikert A, Wilimzig C & Kohne-Volland R (1996). Prophylaxis of migraine with oral magnesium: results from a prospective, multi-center, placebo-controlled and double-blind randomised study. *Cephalalgia* **16**, 257–63.

Pfaffenrath V, Wessely P, Meyer C *et al.* (1996). Magnesium in the prophylaxis of migraine – a double-blind, placebo-controlled study. *Cephalalgia* **16**, 436–40.

Pintov S *et al.* (1997). Acupuncture and the opioid system: implications in management of migraine. *Pediatr Neurol* **17**, 129–33.

Primavera J P & Kaiser R S (1992). Non-pharmacological treatment of headache: is less more? *Headache* **32**, 393–5.

Pryse-Phillips W E M, Dodick D W, Edmeads J G *et al.* (1998). Guidelines for the non-pharmacologic management of migraine in clinical practice. *Can Med Ass J* **159**, 47–54.

Reid G J & McGrath P J (1996). Psychological treatments for migraine. *Biomed Phamacother* **50**, 58–63.

Reilly D (1990). A case of intractable cluster headaches. In *Proceedings of the 1990 professional case conference* (ed. S King, S Kipnis & C Scott). International Foundation for Homoeopathy, Seattle.

Schoenen J, Lenaerts M & Bastings E (1994). High-dose riboflavin as a prophylactic treatment of migraine: results of an open pilot study. *Cephalalgia* **14**, 328–9.

Schoenen J, Jacquy J & Lenaerts M (1998). Effectiveness of high-dose riboflavin in migraine prophylaxis. A randomised controlled trial. *Neurology* **50**, 466–70.

Shekelle P G & Coulter I (1997). Cervical spine manipulation: summary report of a systematic review of the literature and a multidisciplinary expert panel. *J Spinal Dis* **10**, 223–8.

Stodolny J & Chmielewski H (1989). Manual therapy in the treatment of patients with cervical migraine. *J Man Med* **4**, 49–51.

Straumsheim PA, Borchgrevink C, Mowinckel P, Kierulf H & Hafslund O (1997). Homeopatisk behandling av migrene. En dobbelt-blind, placebokontrollert studie av 68 pasienter. *Dynamis* **2**, 18–21.

Tavola T *et al.* (1992). Traditional Chinese acupuncture in tension-type headache: a controlled study. *Pain* **48**, 325–9.

ter Kuile M M, Spinhoven P, Linnsey A C G *et al.* (1994). Autogenic training and cognitive self-hypnosis for the treatment of recurrent headaches in three different subject groups. *Pain* **58**, 331–40.

ter Kuile M M, Spinhoven P & Linssen C G (1995). Responders and non-responders to autogenic training and cognitive self-hypnosis: prediction of short- and long-term success in tension-type headache patients. *Headache* **35**, 630–6.

ter Riet G, Kleijnen J & Knipschild P (1990). Acupuncture and chronic pain: a criteria-based meta-analysis. *J Clin Epidemiol* **11**, 1191–9.

Tisserand R (1985). *The art of aromatherapy.* C W Daniel, Saffron Walden.

VanDyck R, Zitman F G, Linssen A C G & Spinhoven P (1991). Autogenic training and future oriented hypnotic imagery in the treatment of tension headache: outcome and process. *Int J Clin Exp Hypn* **39**, 6–23.

Van Hook E (1998). Non-pharmacological treatment of headaches – why? *Clin Neurosci* **5**, 43–9.

Vernon H T (1989). Spinal manipulation and headaches of cervical origin. *J Manipulative Physiol Ther* **12**, 455–68.

Vernon H (1991). Spinal manipulation and headaches of cervical origin. A review of literature and presentation of cases. *J Man Med* **6**, 73–9.

Vernon H T (1995a). The effectiveness of chiropractic manipulation in the treatment of headache: an exploration of the literature. *J Manipulative Physiol Ther* **18**, 611–17.

Vernon H (1995b). Spinal manipulation and headaches: an update. *Top Clin Chiro* **2**(3), 34–47.

Vincent C A (1989a). A controlled trial of the treatment of migraine by acupuncture. *Clin J Pain* **5**, 305–12.

Vincent C A (1989b). The methodology of controlled trials of acupuncture. *Acup Med* **6**, 9–13.

Vincent C A (1990). The treatment of tension headache by acupuncture: a controlled single case design with time series analysis. *J Psychosom Res* **34**, 553–61.

Vincent C A (1993). Acupuncture as a treatment for chronic pain. In *Clinical research methodology for complementary therapies* (ed. G T Lewith & D Aldridge). Hodder and Stoughton, London.

Vogler BK, Pittler M H & Ernst E (1998). Feverfew as a preventive treatment for migraine: a systematic review. *Cephalalgia* **18**, 704–8.

Walach H, Haeusler W, Lowes T *et al.* (1997). Classical homeopathic treatment of chronic headaches. *Cephalalgia* **17**, 119–26.

White A (1997). Are complementary medicines cost effective? In *Complementary medicine, an objective appraisal* (ed. E Ernst). Butterworth-Heinemann, Oxford.

White A R, Eddleston C, Hardie R, Resch K L & Ernst E (1996). A pilot study of acupuncture for tension headache, using a novel placebo. *Acup Med* **14**, 11–15.

Whitmarsh TE (1997). When conventional treatment is not enough: a case of migraine without aura responding to homoeopathy. *J Alt Comp Med* **3**, 159–62.

Whitmarsh TE, Coleston-Shields DM & Steiner TJ (1997). Double-blind randomized placebo-controlled study of homoeopathic prophylaxis of migraine. *Cephalalgia* **17**, 600–4.

# Index

abdominal migraine  124
absence from work  13, 14–15, 17, 93, 102
acetazolamide  27
acupuncture  128, 131, 136–8
acute infections, as cause of headache  3
adolescents *see* children
adverse events *see* side-effects
age factors  9–10, 12, 46
Alexander technique  149
alternative medicine *see* complementary therapies
amitriptyline  54
anaemia  27
analgesics
　abuse (rebound headache)  34, 36, 38, 46, 55, 64
　children  38
　failed treatment  33
　first-line treatment  35
　second-line treatment  45–6
　as treatment option  32, 33
　withdrawal  55, 65
aneurysms  23, 24
angiography  24
　*see also* magnetic resonance angiography
anticardiolipin antibodies  26
anticoagulant therapy  26, 28, 114
anticonvulsants  29
antidepressants  46, 51, 52, 54
anti-emetics  32, 33, 45, 124
anti-epileptics  46, 131
antihypertensive agents  114
anxiety  52
anxiolytics  131
aromatherapy  149
arterial dissection  27–8
arteriovenous malformations  23, 24–5
aspirin  125

atrioventricular malformation  38
attention deficit disorder  129

basilar migraine  126
behaviour, combative  126
behavioural self-management training  54
benzoic acid  128
berry aneurysm *see* aneurysms
beta-blockers  67, 131
biofeedback  54–5, 131, 147–8
blinded studies  83–4
blindness  28
blood volume pulse  50
blood–brain barrier  69
brain tumours *see* intracranial tumours
breakthrough attacks  33, 36, 66, 67, 69

Cafergot  80, 95–6
calcium-channel blockers  131
carbamazepine  29, 131
carbon monoxide poisoning  37
cardiovascular activity, increased  53
carotid artery, dissection  27–8
cavernous angiomas  25
cerebral hypoxia, as cause of headache  3
cerebral tumours *see* intracranial tumours
cerebrospinal fluid  24, 27
cervical spondylosis  41, 42, 46
cervicogenic headache  139, 140–1
cheese  128, 129
childbirth, traumatic delivery  123
children
　conduct disorders  129
　headache  38, 43, 123
　management  130–2
　medication problems  131
　migraine  123–34
　paramigranous symptoms  124
　placebo response  130

prophylaxis 130–1
sumatriptan 131
tension headache 128
Chinese medicine 136
chiropractic 139–42
chocolate 128
chronic daily headache 36, 54, 63, 64, 65
chronic fatigue syndrome 52–3
City of London Migraine clinic 109
clonidine 118, 130
cluster headache 12, 41, 42, 45, 73
codeine 46, 64
cognitive aspects of headache 49, 52–3
cognitive therapy 54
cold stimulus headache 9
colloid cyst 42
combined oral contraceptive *see* oral contraceptives, combined pill
community pharmacists 34
complementary therapies 32, 135–54
computed tomography (CT)
   arteriovenous malformations 24
   cost-effectiveness 44
   findings 43
   myelography 27
   and raised intracranial pressure 26, 129
   subarachnoid haemorrhage 23–4, 42
   thunderclap headache 42
   unnecessary, hazards 45
   yield 43, 44
conduct disorders 129
confidence intervals 81–3, 87
confusion, episodic 126
consistency studies 83–4
consultation rate 4, 13, 14, 31, 49, 50, 103
cost of illness 13, 13–17
cost–utility analysis 102, 103
cost-effectiveness 31, 101–2
coughing, and headache 42

cow's milk 128
cranial nerve palsies 23
cranial osteopathy 149
cranio-sacral therapy 149
cravings 132
CT *see* computed tomography
cultural factors 49, 50
cyclical vomiting 124
cyproheptadine 130–1

dental diseases, as cause of headache 3
depression
   and acupuncture non-response 128
   and analgesic abuse 46
   and analgesic withdrawal 55
   as cause of headache 46, 51
   and history of abuse 51
   and migraine 49, 52
   and pain 54
dexamethazone 27
diagnosis
   difficulties 46
   by GP 31–2
   reliability 50
diary cards 113
diazepam 131
diclofenac 17, 46
diet and lifestyle
   advice 31
   changes 34
   few foods diet 128–9, 132
   and migraine 127, 128–9, 132, 133
dietary supplements 145–7
direct health care costs 99–101
doctor–patient interaction 54
drugs
   interactions 114
   withdrawal 38
dry needling *see* acupuncture
duplex Doppler sonography 28
dural sinus thrombosis 26

dural tear  27
dysmenorrhoea  112, 114
dysphasia  44

ear diseases, as cause of headache  3
economic effects of headache  12–15
economic evaluation  101
eggs  128
electromyogram biofeedback  147
emotional components of pain  52
endpoints
   calculations  83
   headache relief  77
   headache-free  77
   migraine clinical trials  77–85
   recurrence rate  95
   two-hour response rate  95
epidemiology of headache  3–12
epilepsy  129, 131
epistaxis  125
ergotamine
   abuse  46, 64
   interaction with triptans  72
   in menstrual migraine  112
   in treatment of children  131
   as treatment option  32
erythrocyte sedimentation rate (ESR)  28, 37, 45, 46
ESR *see* erythrocyte sedimentation rate
ethanol  149
eucalyptus oil  149
excitement, as migraine trigger factor  127
extradural haematomas, and intracranial pressure  26
eye disease, as cause of headache  3, 41

facial pain  29, 41
facioplegic migraine  126
falx, meningioma  43
families and friends, effects  3

febrile illness, and headache  123, 129
fenoprofen  114
feverfew (*Tanacetum parthenium*)  131, 148–9
few foods diet  128–9, 132
flurbiprofen  17
focal signs and symptoms  42, 44, 129
food intolerance  145–7
frontal electromyography  50

gabapentin  29
gender factors  5–9, 9, 10, 49, 50, 107
general practice research database (GPRD)  93, 94, 98, 103
general practitioner (GP)
   diagnosis  31–2, 35
   dismissive of symptoms  31, 35
   history taking  31–2, 34, 37
   triptan treatment  70
glaucoma  41
glycerol injections  29
gonadotrophin-releasing hormone  117
growing pains  125

hazard ratio  80
head trauma
   as cause of headache  3
   as trigger factor  128
headache
   *see also* individual types (e.g. migraine, tension headache)
   age factors  5–9, 10, 46
   atypical  26
   causes  3, 23, 36–7, 41, 42, 63
   classification  4–9
      *see also* International Headache Society classification
   consultation rate  4, 13, 14, 31, 49, 50, 103
   and coughing  42
   determinants  3

diagnosis 63–4
differential diagnosis 23–30
effects 3
epidemiology 3–12
familial 51
and febrile illness 123, 129
gender factors 5–9, 49, 50, 107
and hormones 5–9, 46
and intracranial tumours 44–5
investigation 43–4
lifetime history 4
lifetime prevalence 5, 11, 12, 49
long-standing 41
management 34, 35, 36, 42, 65–6
multiple types 6, 35, 38
one-year recall 4
post-traumatic 37
postural 27, 42
prevalence 3–4, 5
as primary symptom 41
progressive history 42–5
prophylaxis 63–76
psychiatric perspectives 49–59
psychogenic 42, 127
psychological factors 52–3
and quality of life 10–12, 35, 52
recurrence 72, 73
self-medication 13
sex distribution *see* gender factors
sexual 25
socioeconomic factors 9, 12–17, 93
subjective nature 4, 50
sudden onset 42
treatment 35, 36, 63–76
triptan therapy 71–2
two-hour response 79
worse in the morning 130
'worst-ever' 38, 41
headache relief as endpoint 77

headache-free as endpoint 77
health visitors 34
hemiparesis 44
hemiplegic migraine 126–7
heparin *see* anticoagulant therapy
history taking
  by GP 31–2, 34, 37
  importance 23
  in outpatient clinic 51
homeopathy 142–5
hormones
  dysfunction 110
  and headache 5–9, 46
  and migraine 107–8, 117–18
  therapeutic use 27, 28, 110, 116–18
Horner's system 27–8
5-HT *see* serotonin
hyperammonaemic syndromes 124
hypertension
  as cause of headache 3, 41
  intracranial 27, 37
hypnotherapy 148
hypoparathyroidism 27
hypotension, intracranial 27
hysterectomy 117

inhaled agents, as trigger factor 128
International Headache Society classification
  cervicogenic headache 139
  in diagnosis 63–4
  major categories 6
  menstrual migraine 109
  migraine 7, 35
  tension headache 7
  trigeminal neuralgia 28–9
intracranial hypertension, benign 27, 41
intracranial pressure, raised 26, 41, 129
intracranial tumours
  *see also* space-occupying lesion
  as cause of headache 3, 41, 44–5

Index **159**

excluding 26, 36–7
and intracranial pressure 26
intraventricular tumour 42
intuition 37, 38

levonorgestrel-releasing intrauterine system, Mirena 116, 118
lifestyle *see* diet
lifetime history of headache 4
lifetime prevalence of headache 5, 11
limb pains, benign 125
lithium 73
liver function tests 124
lumbar puncture 24, 42, 129
lumboperitoneal shunting 27
lupus anticoagulant 26

magnesium 110, 145–6
magnetic resonance (MR)
  angiography 25, 28, 38
  imaging 24, 25, 26, 27
  venography 26
management
  difficulties 45–6
  in primary care 32–4
manipulative therapies 139–42
maple syrup urine disease 124
medical costs of headache 13, 14
  *see also* cost of illness; direct health care costs
medical model of illness 51
Medical Outcomes Study Short Forms SF-20 and SF-36 12
medication
  history 33, 39
  misuse *see* analgesics, abuse
mefenamic acid 114
meningitis 37, 41, 42, 129
menorrhagia 112, 114
menstrual migraine 53, 108–12
  and magnesium 145–6

management 112–14
prophylaxis 114–16
methysergide 131
microvascular decompression 29
migraine
  abdominal 124
  *accompagnée see* migraine, complicated
  acupuncture 128
  aetiology 49
  and anxiety 52
  associated symptoms 83
  attack frequency and duration 31, 63, 93
  attack mechanism 126–7
  average sufferer 31
  childhood 123–34
  classification 7, 35
  and combined oral contraceptive 107–8
  complicated 126, 129, 131
  consultation rate 14, 103
  cost of illness 13–15
  definition 4
  and depression 49, 52
  diagnosis 8, 35, 50, 64, 123
  and diet 127, 128–9, 132, 133
  economic impact 13–15, 17, 93, 102
  and epilepsy 131
  gender factors 107, 126
  heritability 126–7
  homeopathy 143–5
  and hormones 107–8, 117–18
  investigations 129–30
  and magnesium 145–6
  management 36, 65–6, 68–9, 71, 130–2, 150
  menstrual 53, 108–12, 126
  and mood 53
  over-the-counter medication 31
  personality traits 51–2

preconceptions  63
prescription medication  93
prevalence  5, 41, 63, 93, 94, 123
prophylaxis  130–1, 147
and quality of life  31, 39, 55
referral  42
and riboflavin  146–7
socioeconomic factors  50
spinal manipulation  139, 140
and suicidal thoughts  52
termination of attack  79
transformation to chronic form  46
treatment
   clinical effectiveness  77–91
   comparative efficacy  95
   cost-effectiveness  93–105
   options  68–9, 70
   prescription patterns  97–8
   serotonin agonists  17, 65–6
   sumatriptan  17
trigger factors  110, 127–9
in women  107–22
*see also* gender factors
Migraine in Primary Care Advisors (PIPCA) guidelines  32–3
migraine-specific quality of life measure (MSQoL)  55
migranous neuralgia *see* tension headache
Mirena, levonorgestrel-releasing intrauterine system  116, 118
mitochondrial disorders  124, 127
monoamine oxidase inhibitors  73
mood  52, 53
motion sickness  125
mouth ulcers  129
MR *see* magnetic resonance
multidisciplinary management  51, 56
muscular tension  3
*see also* tension headache

nalidixic acid  27
naproxen  114
naratriptan
   *see also* triptans
   cost  98–9
   half-life  72
   headache recurrence  73
   mode of action  69
   trials  96
   two-hour response  72
   well tolerated  85
nausea and vomiting  23, 83, 130
neck stiffness  23
neuroticism  51
nifedipine  131
non-steroidal anti-inflammatory drugs (NSAIDs)  17, 45, 114
*see also specific drugs*
number needed to harm (NNH)  88–9
number needed to treat (NNT)  70, 88–9, 97
Nuprix Pain Report  5

occupational disability, and consultation rate  50
oestradiol  111, 115, 116
oestrogen  111, 114–16, 117
older people, new headache  7, 46
one-year recall of headache  4, 5
open-label studies  83–4
opththalmoplegic migraine  126
optic nerve sheath fenestration  27
oral contraceptives
   combined pill  107–8, 111, 116
   and intracranial hypertension  27
   progestogen-only pill  117
oranges  128
orbital disease  41
organic acidaemia  124
ornithine transcarbamylase deficiency  124

outcome assessment  55
over-the-counter medication  12, 14, 31, 33
  *see also* self-medication
ovulation  110

Paget's disease  41
pain
  chronic  3
  and depression  54
  emotional components  52
  patients' response  50, 51
  subjective  4, 50, 55
  treated by acupuncture  136
papilloedema  27, 42, 44
paramigranous symptoms  124
patient information leaflets  32
patients
  anxieties  41, 45
  compliance  32, 67
  expectations  31, 32, 34, 35–6, 39, 54, 67
  involvement  32, 65–6, 67
  referral demand  35, 38
  relief time important  79, 80
  response to pain  50, 51
  responsibility  38
peppermint oil  149
periodic syndrome  124
personality
  change  44
  traits  51–2
phenobarbitone  131
phenytoin  29, 131
phonophobia  83
photophobia  23, 83
physical exercises  65
physical trigger factors  128
physiotherapy  65
pituitary tumour  42
pizotifen  66–7, 130

placebo effect
  acupuncture  138
  children  38, 130
  clinical trials  79, 80, 87
  enhanced  54
  time course  79
  triptans  87
platelet dysfunction  110
polymyalgia rheumatica  28
population-based studies  3–4
post-traumatic headache  37, 139–40
postural headache  27
practice nurse  34
prescription analysis and cost (PACT)  93, 97, 98
prescription charges  103–4
prescription medication  14, 33, 93, 97–8
primary care
  management decisions  32–4
  records, analysis  94
  referral  31–40
Princess Margaret Migraine Clinic  41–2, 44, 45, 46
progesterone, withdrawal  111
progestogens  116, 117–18
propranolol
  in children  131
  effectiveness  54, 66–7
  for sexual headache  25
  side-effects  67
  trials  66
  and triptans  73
prophylaxis
  agents  66–7
  cost-effectiveness  67, 68
  duration  35–6
  flurbiprofen  17
  guidelines  32–3
  menstrual migraine  114–16
  patient compliance  67

patient expectations 35–6
patient involvement 65–6
surgery 24
as treatment option 32, 45
triptans 114
prostaglandin 112, 114
protein C 26
protein S 26
pseudotumour cerebri 27
psychiatric perspectives 49–59
psychological factors 52–3, 127–8

quality of life
and headache 10–12, 35, 52
importance in diagnosis 63
improving 17
measuring 55
and migraine 31, 39
questionnaire, in GP diagnosis 32

radiosurgery 25, 29
reassurance, premature 45, 51
rebound headache *see* analgesics, abuse
recurrence rate, endpoint 95
referrals
cost-effectiveness 35
effective 39
guidelines 37–8
and medication history 39
patient demand 35, 38
primary care perspective 31–40
secondary care perspective 41–7
to specialist clinic 35–6, 41–2
waiting time 50–1
relaxation training 54–5, 148
relief time, important to patients 79, 80
retrobulbar neuritis (RBN), as cause of headache 41
rhinitis 129
riboflavin 146–7

rizatriptan
*see also* triptans
consistency of response 84
half-life 72
headache recurrence 73
mode of action 69
nausea relief 83
response time 71
trials 80, 96
two-hour response 72
rose-tinted glasses 131
rye 128

school pressures 127
screening, MRI 24
secondary care perspective 41–7
seizures 23, 44, 125
selective serotonin re-uptake inhibitors (SSRIs) 73
self-help techniques 55, 149
self-medication 13, 55
sensory dysfunction 44
sensory migraine 126
serotonin 54, 110
serotonin agonists 17, 63, 65–6, 69, 72
*see also* triptans
sex distribution *see* gender factors
sexual abuse 51, 127
sexual headache 25
side-effects (*general*)
*see also specific drugs*
reporting 84–5
unacceptability 32–3, 34
sinister symptoms *see* headache, causes
sinusitis 41, 42
skin temperature 50
smoking 10
socioeconomic factors 9, 12–17, 50, 93
sodium cromoglycate 145
sodium valproate 131

space-occupying lesion
  *see also* intracranial tumour
  diagnosis  125, 130
specialist clinic, referrals  35–6
statistical analysis of clinical data  81–3
stereotactic radiosurgery  25, 29
steroid treatment  27, 28
stress  53, 127
subarachnoid haemorrhage  23–4, 37, 41, 42
subdural haematomas  26, 42
subjective nature of headache pain  4, 50, 55
suicidal thoughts  52
sumatriptan
  *see also* triptans
  benefits  17
  in children  131
  clinical trials  81, 96
  comparative data  69, 70
  cost  98–9
  efficacy  80, 95–6
  half-life  72
  headache recurrence  73
  market share  97
  mode of action  69
  response time  71
  side-effects  131
  two-hour response  72
survival study methods  80

tartrazine  128
temporal arteritis  28, 37, 41, 42, 45, 46
temporal artery biopsy  28, 37, 45
tension headache
  acupuncture  136–8
  age and sex effects  9–10
  biofeedback prophylaxis  147
  childhood  128
  definition  4
  diagnosis  8, 50, 64

International Headache Society classification  7
  and mood  52
  prevalence  10, 12, 41
  referral  42
  spinal manipulation  139–41
  and stress  53
tetracycline  27
therapeutic gain  70, 85–7
thermal biofeedback  147
thunderclap headache  24, 42
*tic douloureux see* trigeminal neuralgia
tinnitus  27
tolfenamic acid  95–6
tomatoes  128
torticollis, benign paroxysmal  125
transcendental meditation  148
transient ischaemic attack  27–8
treatment
  costs  94
  failure  33–4, 35, 45
  options  32, 45–6
  second-line  45–6
  successful  53–4
tricyclic antidepressants  54
  *see also* antidepressants
trigeminal neuralgia  28–9, 41, 46
trigger factors
  avoidance  69
  childhood migraine  127–9
  food intolerance  145–7
  menstrual  110, 112
  non-hormonal  113
trigger points, myofascial  136
triptans
  in children  38
  comparison  96–7
  costs and cost-effectiveness  35, 45, 98–101
  efficacy  95
  failed treatment  34

formulations  69
interactions  72, 73
mode of action  69
NHS funding  102–4
placebo response in trials  87
in primary care  70
prophylactic  114
safety  85
selection  69–73
as treatment option  32, 33
trials  96–7
two-hour response  87–8
two-hour response rate, as endpoint  95

uveitis  41

vaginal discharge  129
verapamil  131
vertebral artery, dissection  28
vertigo, benign paroxysmal  125
visual field defects  44
visual symptoms  27
vitamin A toxicity  27
vomiting *see* nausea and vomiting

warfarin *see* anticoagulant therapy
weather conditions, as trigger factor  128
wheat  128
women *see* gender factors; menstrual migraine
work lost *see* absence from work; socioeconomic factors
'worst-ever' headache  38, 41

xanthochromia  24

York Headache Clinic  35, 38

zolmitriptan
  *see also* triptans
  dose–response relationship  82, 85, 86
  half-life  72
  headache recurrence  73
  mode of action  69
  trials  96
  two-hour response  72